High-Yield Lung

High-Yield Systems
High-Yield Lung

Ronald W. Dudek, PhD
Brody School of Medicine
East Carolina University
Department of Anatomy and Cell Biology
Greenville, North Carolina

LIPPINCOTT WILLIAMS & WILKINS
A **Wolters Kluwer** Company

Philadelphia • Baltimore • New York • London
Buenos Aires • Hong Kong • Sydney • Tokyo

Acquisitions Editor: Betty Sun
Managing Editor: Elena Coler
Marketing Manager: Emilie Linkins
Production Editor: Jennifer D. W. Glazer
Designer: Terry Mallon
Compositor: Circle Graphics, Inc
Printer: Courier—Kendallville

351 West Camden Street
Baltimore, MD 21201

530 Walnut Street
Philadelphia, PA 19106

Printed in the United States of America

Library of Congress Cataloging-in-Publication Data

Dudek, Ronald W., 1950-
    High-yield lung / Ronald W. Dudek.—1st ed.
       p. ; cm.—(High-yield systems)
    Includes index.
    ISBN 0-7817-5570-0
    1. Lungs—Pathophysiology—Outlines, syllabi, etc. 2. Lungs—Outlines, syllabi, etc. 3. Medical sciences—Outlines, syllabi, etc. 4. Physicians—Licenses—United States—Examinations—Study guides.
I. Title. II. Series.
    [DNLM: 1. Lung—Examination Questions. 2. Lung Diseases—Examination Questions. WF 18.2
D845h 2006]
RC756.D83 2006
616.2′4′0076—dc22

                                                                                    2005009801

To purchase additional copies of this book, call our customer service department at **(800) 638-3030** or fax orders to **(301) 824-7390**. International customers should call **(301) 714-2324**.

Visit Lippincott Williams & Wilkins on the Internet: http://www.LWW.com. Lippincott Williams & Wilkins customer service representatives are available from 8:30 am to 6:00 pm, EST.

                                        05 06 07 08 09
                                        1 2 3 4 5 6 7 8 9 10

Preface

A focused curriculum is a curriculum whereby students are immersed in one basic science discipline (e.g., histology) for a concentrated period of time, during which histology is covered from A to Z. A systems-based curriculum is a curriculum whereby students are immersed in one system (e.g., respiratory system) for a concentrated period of time, during which all basic science disciplines of the respiratory system are covered (e.g., embryology, histology, physiology, pharmacology, and so forth).

The High-Yield Systems Series addresses a problem endemic to medical schools in the United States and medical students using a focused curriculum. After completing a focused curriculum, the medical student is faced with the daunting task of integrating and collating all the basic science knowledge accrued from the focused curriculum into the various systems. For example, a medical student wanting to review everything about the lung will find the information scattered in his/her embryology notes, histology notes, physiology notes, pharmacology notes, and so forth. The High-Yield Systems Series eliminates this daunting task for the medical student by bringing together the embryology, gross anatomy, radiology, histology, physiology, microbiology, and pharmacology of the lung in one clear and concise book.

The High-Yield Systems Series is useful for the following:

1. First-year medical students in a focused curriculum who want to get a head-start on the inevitable integration and collation process of all the information learned in a focused curriculum into systems.
2. First-year medical students in a systems-based curriculum will find this series a natural textbook for a systems-based curriculum.
3. Medical students preparing for Step 1 of the USMLE, in which the questions are becoming increasingly more systems- than discipline-based.
4. Second-year medical students in which the curriculum is much more systems-based, as pathology covers the pathology of each system as a block (e.g., pathology of the lung, pathology of the heart, pathology of the kidney, etc.).
5. Senior medical students may want to quickly review all aspects of lung function before starting a rotation in pulmonology, for example.
6. Recent medical graduates may want to quickly review all aspects of lung function before starting a residency in pulmonology, for example.

In the High-Yield Systems Series, the student will find the same painstaking attention given to include high-yield information as found in other High-Yield books. However, the breadth of information has been expanded somewhat to cover some baseline information without which a complete understanding of the system would be difficult.

The High-Yield books, based on the presentation of high-yield information that is likely to be asked on the USMLE, have clearly been an asset to the medical student. However, after writing many High-Yield books, I have found that high-yield information can also be presented in a high-efficiency manner. In the High-Yield Systems Series, the student now gets the benefit of both high yield and high efficiency in their studies.

I appreciate any feedback and can be contacted at dudekr@mail.ecu.edu.

Table of Contents

Chapter 1

Embryology of the Lung

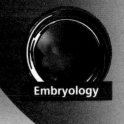

Embryology

❶ General Features

The respiratory system is divided into the **upper and lower respiratory systems.** The upper respiratory system consists of the **nose, nasopharynx,** and **oropharynx** and is typically discussed with head and neck embryology, namely the pharyngeal apparatus. The lower respiratory system (*Fig. 1-1*) consists of the **larynx, trachea, bronchi,** and **lungs.** The first sign of development is the formation of the **respiratory diverticulum** in the ventral wall of the primitive **foregut** during week 4, both of which are lined by **endoderm** and surrounded by a bed of **mesoderm.** The distal end of the respiratory diverticulum enlarges to form the **lung bud.** The lung bud divides into two **bronchial buds** that branch into the **main (primary), lobar (secondary), segmental (tertiary),** and **subsegmental bronchi.** The respiratory diverticulum initially is in open communication with the foregut, but eventually they become separated by indentations of mesoderm, the **tracheoesophageal folds.** When the tracheoesophageal folds fuse in the midline to form the **tracheoesophageal septum,** the foregut is divided into the trachea ventrally and the esophagus dorsally. The **Hox-complex, FGF-10** (fibroblast growth factor), **BMP-4** (bone morphogenetic protein), **N-*myc*** (a proto-oncogene), **syndecan** (a proteoglycan), **tenascin** (an extracellular matrix protein), and **epimorphin** (a protein) appear to play a role in development of the respiratory system.

[margin handwritten notes: Hox / FgF-10 / BMP-4 / N myc / Syndecan / tenascin / epimorphin]

❷ Development of the Larynx

The opening of the respiratory diverticulum into the foregut becomes the **laryngeal orifice.** The laryngeal epithelium and glands are derived from endoderm. The laryngeal muscles are derived from somitomeric mesoderm of pharyngeal arches 4 and 6 and therefore are innervated by branches of the vagus nerve (CN X); that is, the superior laryngeal nerve and recurrent laryngeal nerve, respectively. The laryngeal cartilages (thyroid, cricoid, arytenoid, corniculate, and cuneiform) are also derived from somitomeric mesoderm of pharyngeal arches 4 and 6.

[margin handwritten note: Arch 4+6]

❸ Development of the Trachea

A. **Sources.** The tracheal epithelium and glands are derived from endoderm. The tracheal smooth muscle, connective tissue, and C-shaped cartilage rings are derived from mesoderm.

B. **Clinical considerations of the trachea**
   1. A **tracheoesophageal fistula** is an abnormal communication between the trachea and esophagus that results from improper division of foregut by the tracheoesophageal septum. It is generally associated with **esophageal atresia** and **polyhydramnios.** Clinical features include: excessive accumulation of saliva or mucus in the nose and mouth; episodes of gagging and cyanosis after swallowing milk; abdominal distension after crying; and reflux of gastric contents into the lungs, causing pneumonitis. Diagnostic features include: inability to pass a catheter into the stomach and radiographs demonstrating air in the infant's stomach.
   2. **Tracheal agenesis** is a rare congenital abnormality that may occur in three forms. **In Type I,** the upper trachea is absent while the lower trachea is connected to the esophagus. **In Type II,** the trachea is absent while a common bronchus that branches

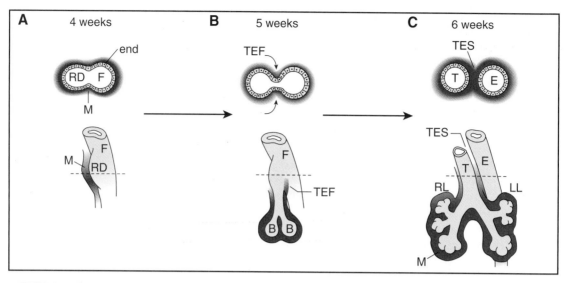

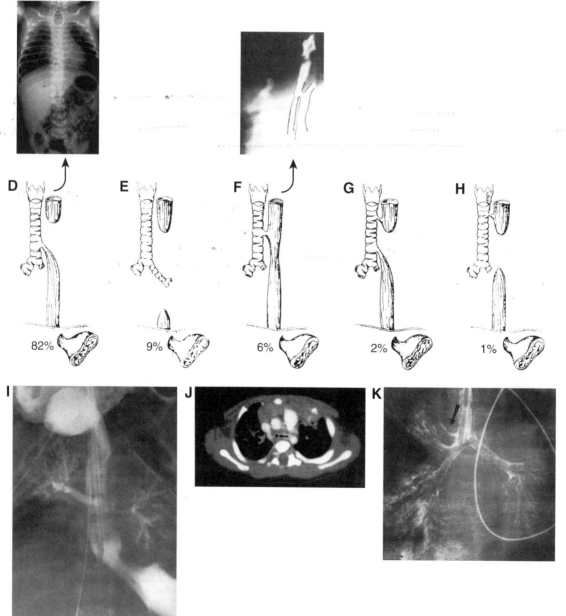

into a right and left main bronchus arises from the esophagus. **In Type III,** the right and left main bronchi arise from the esophagus. Clinical features include: immediate, severe respiratory distress, absence of a cry, and inability to intubate below the larynx.

3. **Tracheal stenosis** is a rare congenital abnormality caused by the complete lack of cartilaginous rings in the tracheal wall resulting in a narrowing of the tracheal lumen. Acquired tracheal stenosis usually is caused by intubation or traumatic tracheobronchial suctioning.

4. **Tracheal bronchus** occurs when an ectopic bronchus branches directly from the trachea. This generally occurs on the right so that the tracheal bronchus supplies the entire right upper lobe or an apical bronchopulmonary segment. Sometimes, a supernumerary segment may be present.

5. **Tracheomalacia** is a rare congenital abnormality caused by the softening of the cartilaginous rings in the tracheal wall. Clinical features include: expiratory stridor (wheezing) during crying, reflex apnea ("dying spells"), and sometimes cyanosis/bradycardia after feeding.

Ⅳ Development of the Bronchi

A. **Stages of development.** The lung bud divides into two **bronchial buds.** In week 5 of development, bronchial buds enlarge to form **main (primary) bronchi.** The right main bronchus is larger and more vertical than the left main bronchus. This relationship persists throughout adult life and accounts for the greater likelihood of foreign bodies lodging on the right side than on the left. The main bronchi further subdivide into **lobar (secondary) bronchi** (3 on the right side and 2 on the left side, corresponding to the lobes of the adult lung). The lobar bronchi further subdivide into **segmental (tertiary) bronchi** (10 on the right side and 9 on the left side), which further subdivide into **subsegmental bronchi.** The segmental bronchi are the primordia of the **bronchopulmonary segments,** which are morphologically and functionally separate respiratory units of the lung. As the endoderm-lined bronchi continue to branch into the bed of mesoderm, the airways become progressively smaller and expand into a space known as the primitive pleural cavity. The mesoderm covering the surface of the lung develops into **visceral pleura,** and somatic mesoderm covering the inside of the body wall develops into **parietal pleura.** The space between the visceral and parietal pleura is called the **pleural cavity.**

◀

FIGURE 1-1. Development of the respiratory system at (A) 4 weeks, (B) 5 weeks, and (C) 6 weeks. Both lateral views and cross-sectional views are shown. Note the relationship of the respiratory diverticulum (*RD*) and foregut (*F*), both of which are lined by endoderm and surrounded by a bed of mesoderm (*M*). Note that as the endoderm-lined bronchi continue to branch into the bed of mesoderm, the airways become progressively smaller. This branching is controlled by cell interactions between the endoderm and mesoderm called epithelio-mesenchymal interactions. *Curved arrows* indicate the movement of the tracheoesophageal folds (*TEF*) as the tracheoesophageal septum (*TES*) forms between the trachea (*T*) and esophagus (*E*). B—bronchial buds; RL—right lung; LL—left lung. **(D–H) Five different anatomical types of esophagus and trachea malformations. (D)** Esophageal atresia with a tracheoesophageal fistula at the distal one-third end of the trachea. This is the most common type, occurring in 82% of cases. The AP radiograph of this malformation shows an enteric tube (*arrow*) coiled in the upper esophageal pouch. The air in the bowel indicates a distal tracheoesophageal fistula. **(E)** Esophageal atresia only, occurring in 9% of cases. **(F)** H-type tracheoesophageal fistula only, occurring in 6% of cases. The barium swallow radiograph shows a normal esophagus (*E*), but dye has spilled into the trachea (*T*) through the fistula and outlines the upper trachea and larynx. **(G)** Esophageal atresia with a tracheoesophageal fistula at both proximal and distal ends, occurring in 2% of cases. **(H)** Esophageal atresia with a tracheoesophageal fistula at the proximal end, occurring in 1% of cases. **(I) Type II tracheal agenesis.** Postmortem AP esophagogram of a term newborn with severe respiratory distress. Note the common bronchus arising from the esophagus. **(J) Tracheal stenosis.** A CT scan shows severe narrowing of the lumen of the trachea. Note that the lumen of the trachea is a "perfect circle" rather than oval-shaped. **(K) Tracheal bronchus.** A tracheogram shows a right tracheal bronchus (*arrow*) along with a collapsed right upper lobe.

B. Sources. The bronchial epithelium and glands are derived from endoderm. The bronchial smooth muscle, connective tissue, and cartilage are derived from mesoderm.

C. Clinical considerations of the bronchi *(Fig. 1-2)*

1. The **bronchopulmonary segment** is a segment of lung tissue supplied by a **segmental (tertiary) bronchus, a branch of the pulmonary artery, a branch of the bronchial artery, and a branch of the bronchial vein,** all of which run through the **center** of the bronchopulmonary segment. **Branches of the pulmonary veins** are found at the **periphery** between two adjacent bronchopulmonary segments (i.e., intersegmental location), which form **surgical landmarks** during segmental resection. Surgeons can resect diseased lung tissue along bronchopulmonary segments instead of removing the entire lobe.

2. **Congenital lobar emphysema (CLE)** is characterized by progressive overdistension of one of the upper lobes or the right middle lobe with **air.** The term emphysema is a misnomer, as there is no destruction of the alveolar walls. Although the exact etiology remains unknown, many cases involve **collapsed bronchi** as a result of **failure of bronchial cartilage formation.** In this situation, air can be inspired through collapsed bronchi but cannot be expired. During the first few days of life, fluid may be trapped in the involved lobe, producing an opaque, enlarged hemithorax. Later, the fluid is resorbed and the classic radiological appearance of an emphysematous **(air-filled)** lobe with generalized radiolucency (hyperlucent) is apparent.

3. **Congenital bronchogenic cysts** represent an abnormality in bronchial branching and may be found within the mediastinum (most commonly around the carina, upper trachea, or main bronchi) or intrapulmonary. Intrapulmonary cysts are round, solitary, sharply marginated, **fluid-filled,** and do not initially communicate with the tracheobronchial tree. Cysts are lined by a ciliated epithelium and have smooth muscle and cartilage in its wall. Because intrapulmonary bronchogenic cysts contain fluid, they appear as water-density masses on chest radiographs. These cysts may become air-filled as a result of infection or instrumentation.

4. **Congenital cystic adenomatous malformation** is a hamartomatous proliferation of terminal bronchioles at the expense of alveoli, which results in both cysts and solid masses. The cysts are lined by an adenomatous epithelium and communicate with the rest of the tracheobronchial tree.

5. **Pulmonary sequestration** occurs when a mass of pulmonary tissue forms that is not connected to the tracheobronchial tree or pulmonary artery. If the pulmonary mass is located within the lung, it is called an **intralobar sequestration (ILS).** An ILS usually occurs in the lower lobes, is supplied by an anomalous artery branching from the aorta, and is drained by the pulmonary veins. If the pulmonary mass is located outside the lung, it is called an extralobar sequestration (ELS). An ELS usually occurs on the left side between the lower lobe and the diaphragm, is supplied by an anomalous artery branching from the aorta, and is drained by the azygous vein.

▶

FIGURE 1-2. (A) Distribution of bronchopulmonary segments and their relationship to the tracheobronchial tree. Segmental bronchi of the right and left lungs are numbered. *Right Lung:* 1,2,3: segmental bronchi that branch from the upper lobar bronchus; 4,5: segmental bronchi that branch from the middle lobar bronchus; 6,7,8,9,10: segmental bronchi that branch from the lower lobar bronchus. Note that bronchopulmonary segment #7 is not represented on the outer costal surface of the right lung (#7 is located on the inner mediastinal surface). *Left Lung:* 1,2,3,4,5: segmental bronchi that branch from the upper lobar bronchus; 6,8,9,10: segmental bronchi that branch from the lower lobar bronchus. Note that there is no #7 segmental bronchus associated with the left lung. **(B) Congenital lobar emphysema.** Expiratory AP radiograph shows a hyperlucent area in the emphysematous right upper lobe caused by air trapping. The affected lobe is overdistended and the mediastinum may be shifted to the contralateral side. Secondary ipsilateral compression of the lower lobe or herniation of the upper lobe into the mediastinum may occur. **(C) Congenital bronchogenic cyst.** AP radiograph shows a large, opaque area in the right upper lobe, caused by an intrapulmonary fluid-filled cyst. **(d) intrathoracic bronchogenic cyst.** CT scan shows an intrathoracic bronchogenic cyst (*C*) located near the carina. **(E) Congenital cystic adenomatous malformation.** CT scan shows a complex cystic mass in the right lower lobe with a reticulated, bubbly appearance. **(F, G) Pulmonary sequestration.** CT scan shows an extrapulmonary sequestration whereby a pulmonary mass (*arrowheads*) is present, associated with the left lower lobe. A pulmonary arteriogram shows an anomalous artery branching from the aorta to supply the sequestration.

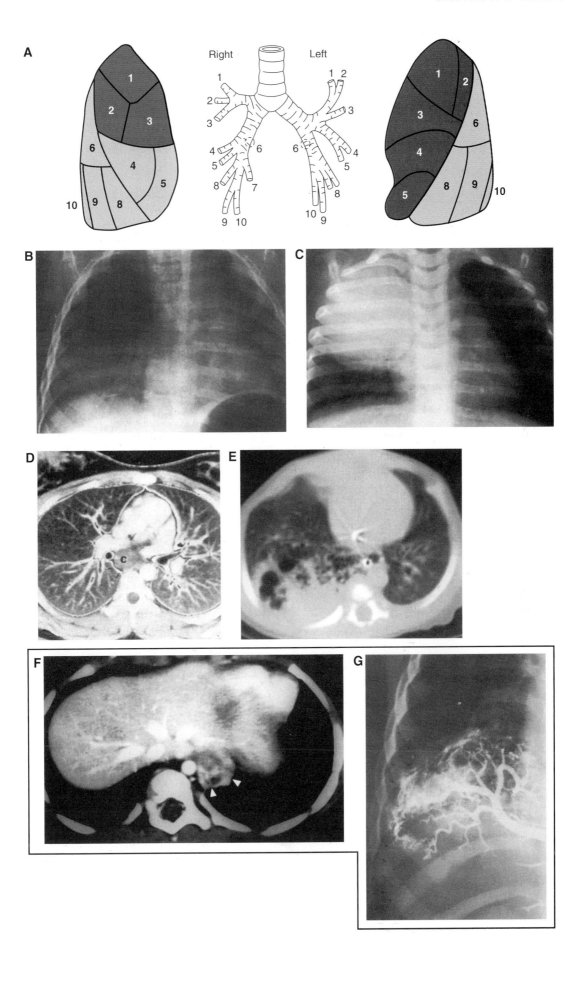

6. A **bronchoesophageal fistula** is an abnormal communication between a bronchus and the esophagus, which usually is found on the right side in association with esophageal atresia.

7. **Bronchial atresia** is an abnormal closure of either lobar bronchi or segmental bronchi usually of the upper lobe. At birth, the obstructed lung may be filled with fluid and thus appear as a pulmonary mass. Later, the fluid is resorbed and replaced by air such that the lung becomes emphysematous. A central, oval, or fan-shaped accumulation of mucus distal to the obstruction (called a **mucocele**) may be present.

Ⓥ Development of the Lungs

A. **Periods of development** *(Fig. 1-3)*. The lung matures in a proximal–distal direction, beginning with the largest bronchi and proceeding outward. As a result, lung development is heterogeneous; proximal pulmonary tissue will be in a more advanced period of development than distal pulmonary tissue.

1. **Pseudoglandular period (weeks 7–16).** During this period, the developing lung resembles an exocrine gland. The numerous **endodermal tubules** are lined by sim-

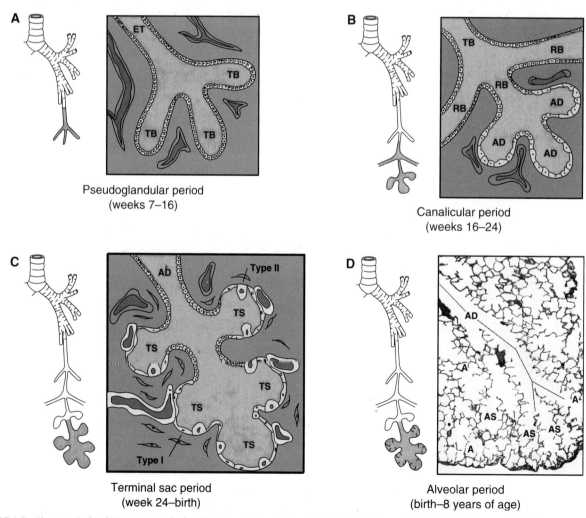

FIGURE 1-3. Time periods of lung development. (A) Pseudoglandular period, **(B)** Canalicular period, **(C)** Terminal sac period, **(D)** Alveolar period. ET—endodermal tubules; TB—terminal bronchiole; RB—respiratory bronchiole; AD—alveolar duct; TS—terminal sac; AS—alveolar sac; A—alveoli.

ple columnar epithelium that give rise to the epithelium of the future airways and are surrounded by **mesoderm** that give rise to the future connective tissue components of the lung (i.e., cartilage, collagen and elastic fibers, smooth muscle and vasculature). At this time period, the mesoderm forms only a **modest capillary network.** Each endodermal tubule branches into **15–25 terminal bronchioles.** During this period, respiration is not possible and premature infants cannot survive.

2. **Canalicular period (weeks 16–24).** During this period, the terminal bronchioles branch into three or more **respiratory bronchioles.** The respiratory bronchioles subsequently branch into 3 to 6 **alveolar ducts.** The terminal bronchioles, respiratory bronchioles, and alveolar ducts are now lined by a **simple cuboidal epithelium** and are surrounded by mesoderm containing a **prominent capillary network.** Premature infants born before week 20 rarely survive.

3. **Terminal sac period (week 24–birth).** During this period, **terminal sacs** bud off the alveolar ducts and then dilate and expand into the surrounding mesoderm. The terminal sacs are separated from each other by **primary septae.** The simple cuboidal epithelium within the terminal sacs differentiates into **type I pneumocytes** (thin, flat cells that make up part of the blood-air barrier) and **type II pneumocytes** (which produce surfactant). The terminal sacs are surrounded by mesoderm containing a **rapidly proliferating capillary network.** The capillaries make intimate contact with the terminal sacs and thereby establish a **blood-air barrier** with the type I pneumocytes. **Premature infants born between week 25 and week 28 can survive** with intensive care. Adequate vascularization and surfactant levels are the most important factors for the survival of premature infants.

4. **Alveolar period (birth–8 years of age).** During this period, terminal sacs are partitioned by **secondary septae** to form adult **alveoli.** Approximately 20 to 70 million alveoli are present at birth. Approximately 300 to 400 million alveoli are present by 8 years of age. The major mechanism for the increase in the number of alveoli is formation of secondary septae that partition existing alveoli. After birth, the increase in the size of the lung is the result of an **increase in the number of respiratory bronchioles.** The diameter of the pulmonary acinus (all airways distal to the terminal bronchiole) is **1 to 2 mm** at birth and gradually increases to its adult diameter of **6 to 10 mm** by adolescence. On chest radiographs, lungs of a newborn infant are denser than those of an adult lung because of the fewer number of mature alveoli.

B. **Clinical considerations of the lung** (Fig. 1-4)
1. **Retained fluid syndrome (or "wet lung disease")** is caused by delayed resorption and clearance of lung fluid and is one of the most common causes of respiratory distress in the newborn. Clinical features include: tachypnea, nasal flaring, grunting, and retractions. Radiographic findings include: fluid within the lungs, parahilar radiating congestion, vascular markings with hazy borders, and fluid within fissures. The lungs generally begin to clear within 10 to 12 hours. **Aeration at birth** is the replacement of lung liquid with air in the newborn's lungs. In the fetal state, the functional residual capacity (FRC) of the lung is filled with liquid secreted by fetal lung epithelium (up to 500 mL/day) via Cl⁻ transport using **CFTR (cystic fibrosis transmembrane protein)** and **CIC-2 (volume-activated chloride channel.** At birth, lung liquid is eliminated by a reduction in lung liquid secretion via Na⁺ transport (H₂O follows) by type II pneumocytes and resorption into pulmonary capillaries (major route) and lymphatics (minor route). Lungs of a stillborn baby will sink when placed in water because they contain fluid rather than air.

2. **Respiratory distress syndrome (RDS)** is caused by a deficiency or absence of **surfactant.** This surface active agent is composed of **cholesterol (50%), dipalmitoylphosphatidylcholine** (DPPC; 40%), and **surfactant proteins A, B, and C (10%)** and coats the inside of alveoli to maintain alveolar patency. RDS is prevalent in: premature infants (accounts for 50–70% of deaths in premature infants),

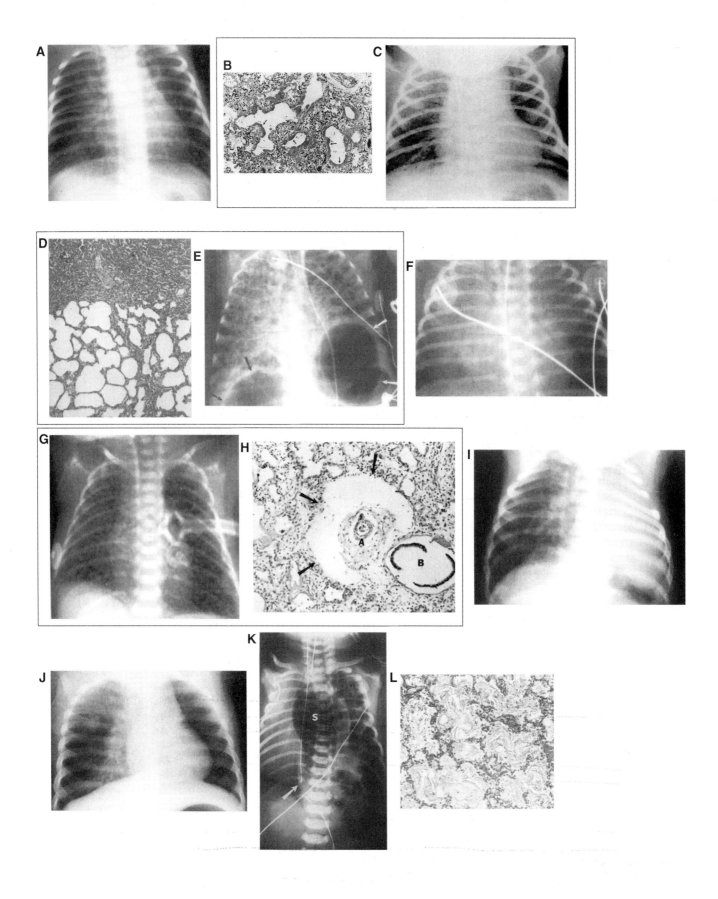

infants of diabetic mothers, infants who experienced fetal asphyxia or maternofetal hemorrhage (damages type II pneumocytes), and multiple birth infants. Clinical features include: dyspnea, tachypnea, inspiratory retractions of the chest wall, expiratory grunting, cyanosis, and nasal flaring. Treatments include: administration of betamethasone (a corticosteroid) to the mother for several days before delivery (i.e., antenatal) to increase surfactant production, postnatal administration of an artificial surfactant solution, and postnatal high-frequency ventilation. RDS in premature infants cannot be discussed without mentioning **germinal matrix hemorrhage (GMH).** The germinal matrix is the site of proliferation of neuronal and glial precursors in the developing brain, which is located above the caudate nucleus, in the floor of the lateral ventricles, and the caudothalamic groove. The germinal matrix also contains a rich network of fragile, thin-walled blood vessels. The brain of the premature infant lacks the ability to autoregulate the cerebral blood pressure. Consequently, increased arterial blood pressure in these blood vessels leads to rupture and hemorrhage into the germinal matrix. This leads to significant neurologic sequelae, including cerebral palsy, mental retardation, and seizures. Antenatal corticosteroid administration has a clear role in reducing the incidence of GMH in premature infants.

3. **Bronchopulmonary dysplasia (BPD)** occurs when infants with respiratory distress syndrome are placed on O_2 and positive-pressure ventilation. High concentrations of O_2 (i.e., O_2 toxicity) damage the basement membrane of pulmonary arterioles, leading to leaky lung syndrome. Positive-pressure ventilation causes mechanical damage leading to "bubbly lungs." The "bubbly lungs" result from hyperaeration of some alveoli and atelectasis of other alveoli. Radiographic findings include: haziness of blood vessel margins during week 1–2 of life which progresses to linear densities that persist into week 3–4 of life; gradual appearance of "bubbly lungs," whose appearance is quite variable but generally pronounced at the bases; some infants may develop large pneumatoceles. Long-term BPD leads to submucosal fibrosis of bronchi, septal fibrosis, chronic inflammation, and squamous metaplasia of terminal bronchioles and alveoli.

4. **Wilson-Mikity syndrome** is a condition very similar to BPD (see above) and indeed some clinicians consider them to be the same disease. Classic Wilson-Mikity syndrome occurs when infants with initially clear lungs (i.e., no apparent respiratory distress) develop "bubbly lungs."

5. **Leaky lung syndrome** occurs when infants with respiratory distress syndrome are placed on O_2 and positive-pressure ventilation. O_2 toxicity damages the basement

◀

FIGURE 1-4. (A) Retained fluid syndrome (RFS). AP radiograph shows pronounced bilateral parahilar infiltrates with some fluid in the minor fissure. **(B and C) Respiratory distress syndrome (RDS).** *Light micrograph.* The pathological hallmarks are acinar atelectasis (i.e., collapse of the respiratory acinus, which includes the respiratory bronchioles, alveolar ducts, and alveoli), dilation of terminal bronchioles (*), and deposition of an eosinophilic hyaline membrane material (*arrows*) that consists of fibrin and necrotic cells. *AP radiograph.* The radiological hallmarks are a bell-shaped thorax caused by underaeration and reticulogranularity of the lungs caused by acinar atelectasis. **(D and E) Bronchopulmonary dysplasia (BPD).** Light micrograph shows alternating areas of hyperaeration and atelectasis causing a "bubbly lung" appearance. AP radiograph shows predominately the "bubbly lung" appearance along with two large pneumatoceles (*arrows*). **(F) Leaky lung syndrome.** AP radiograph shows that the lungs are opaque and hazy. The lungs are larger in size as a result of the edema than when the respiratory distress occurred initially. **(G and H) Pulmonary air leaks.** AP radiograph shows a typical salt-and-pepper appearance of pulmonary interstitial emphysema (PIE) as a result of the radiolucent air surrounding bronchovascular sheaths. Note the left chest tube that was placed to treat the pneumothorax. Light micrograph shows the escaped air (arrows) surrounding the bronchovascular sheath. A—pulmonary arteriole; B—bronchiole. **(I) Unilateral pulmonary agenesis.** AP radiograph shows complete absence of the left lung with a shift of the mediastinum to the left hemithorax. In addition, the right lung shows hypervascularity and overdistension. **(J) Unilateral pulmonary hypoplasia.** AP radiograph shows decreased size of the left lung with a shift of the mediastinum to the left hemithorax. In addition, the right lung shows hypervascularity. **(K) Congenital diaphragmatic hernia.** aP radiograph shows air-filled stomach (S) and air-filled loops of intestine in the left hemithorax with a shift of the mediastinum to the right hemithorax. Note the tip of the nasogastric tube is in the distal esophagus (*arrow*). **(L) Meconium aspiration syndrome.** Light micrograph shows meconium with a large number of epithelial squames within the terminal airways and alveoli.

membrane of pulmonary arterioles, leading to leakage of fluid initially into the pulmonary interstitium and then intra-alveolar. This results in pulmonary edema, which is one of the most common abnormalities seen in premature infants.

6. **Pulmonary air leaks** occur when terminal airways and alveoli become overdistended with air and rupture, most commonly caused by positive-pressure ventilation. The air escapes into the pulmonary interstitium, causing a serious condition called **pulmonary interstitial emphysema (PIE).** The air tracts along the bronchovascular sheaths (some believe the air is intralymphatic) radiating to the outer periphery of the lung. The air may burst into the mediastinum, pleural cavity, or pericardial cavity, resulting in **pneumomediastinum, pneumothorax,** or **pneumopericardium,** respectively.

7. **Pulmonary agenesis** is the complete absence of a lung or a lobe and its bronchi. This is a rare condition caused by failure of bronchial buds to develop. Unilateral pulmonary agenesis is compatible with life.

8. **Pulmonary aplasia** is the absence of lung tissue but the presence of a rudimentary bronchus.

9. **Pulmonary hypoplasia (PH) is** a poorly developed bronchial tree with abnormal histology. PH classically involves the right lung in association with right-sided obstructive congenital heart defects. PH can also be found in association with **congenital diaphragmatic hernia** (see below), which compresses the developing lung. PH can also be found in association with **bilateral renal agenesis,** which causes an insufficient amount of amniotic fluid (oligohydramnios) to be produced, which in turn increases pressure on the fetal thorax.

10. A **congenital diaphragmatic hernia** is a herniation of abdominal contents into the pleural space, caused by a failure of the **pleuroperitoneal membrane** to develop or fuse with the other components of the diaphragm. The hernia most commonly occurs through the **left posterior pleuroperitoneal canal (Bochdalek hernia).** The hernia is usually life-threatening because abdominal contents compress the bronchial buds and cause pulmonary hypoplasia. A serious complication that occurs is **persistent pulmonary hypertension.** Clinical signs in the newborn include: unusually flat abdomen, breathlessness, and cyanosis.

11. **Meconium aspiration syndrome** is the intrauterine or intrapartum aspiration of meconium-stained amniotic fluid, most commonly caused by fetal distress, whereby meconium is released into the amniotic fluid and fetal gasping occurs. Meconium is a viscous, greenish-black material that contains: mucus, epithelial squames, bile, and other swallowed material like lanugo hairs.

12. **Congenital pulmonary lymphangiectasis (CPL)** is a rare condition that involves impaired lymph drainage from the lung. If CPL is an isolated abnormality, it is most likely caused by arrest of lymphatic vessel development along with the persistence of dilated and obstructed lymphatic vessels. CPL may also occur in conjunction with some congenital heart defects that result in increased pulmonary venous obstruction (e.g., hypoplastic left heart syndrome).

13. **Chylothorax** is the accumulation of a large amount of lymph in the pleural space, the etiology of which is uncertain although traumatic tears in the thoracic duct during delivery have been implicated. The lymph does not become chylous until milk or formula feeding begins.

14. **Horseshoe lung** is a rare anomaly whereby part of the left lower lobe of the lung is located ectopically posterior to the heart and joins the right lower lobe of the lung.

Ⅵ Development of the Pulmonary Vascular System

The adult lung is supplied by two arterial systems and drained by two venous systems.

A. The **pulmonary trunk** is derived from one of the five dilatations of the primitive heart tube, namely the **truncus arteriosus,** which is divided into the aorta and pulmonary trunk by the **aorticopulmonary septum.** The **proximal parts of the right and left pulmonary arteries** are derived from the **right and left sixth aortic arches.** The **smaller** intraparenchymal branches of the pulmonary arteries are derived from the **mesodermal bed surrounding the airways,** which forms an arterial network alongside the airways. As the airways branch, the pulmonary arteries branch to follow the airways to the level of the terminal bronchioles, at which point they form a capillary plexus. This explains the adult relationship whereby branches of the airways track along with branches of the pulmonary arteries. (Note: In the adult, airways track along with branches of the pulmonary arteries, bronchial arteries, and bronchial veins; see below).

B. The **primitive bronchial arteries** form early in embryonic development from the aorta near the celiac trunk but later disappear. The **one definitive right bronchial artery** is derived as a branch of the **posterior intercostal artery** and the **two definitive left bronchial arteries** are derived as branches from the **thoracic aorta.** The **smaller intraparenchymal branches of the bronchial arteries** are derived from the **mesodermal bed surrounding the airways,** which forms an arterial network alongside the airways. As the airways branch, the bronchial arteries branch to follow the airways to the level of the terminal bronchioles. This explains the adult relationship whereby branches of the airways track along with branches of the bronchial arteries.

C. The **common pulmonary vein** develops as an outgrowth of the dorsal wall of the **left atrium** and establishes a connection to the pulmonary vascular bed, which drains via **four pulmonary veins.** As the left atrium grows, the transient common pulmonary vein is incorporated into the wall of the left atrium, forming the smooth part of the left atrium. As a result, the four pulmonary veins empty directly into the left atrium. The **smaller intraparenchymal branches of the pulmonary veins** are derived from the **mesodermal bed NOT surrounding the airways,** which forms a venous network in solo within the interstitium of the lung. This explains the adult relationship whereby branches of the pulmonary veins lie alone within the interstitium of the lung.

D. The **right bronchial vein** is derived as a branch of the **azygos vein** and the **left bronchial vein** is derived as a branch of the **accessory hemiazygos vein.** The azygous system of veins forms embryologically from the **supracardinal system** of veins. The **smaller intraparenchymal branches of the bronchial veins** are derived from the **mesodermal bed surrounding the airways,** which forms a venous network alongside the airways in association with the bronchial arteries. This explains the adult relationship whereby branches of the airways track along with branches of the bronchial veins.

E. **Clinical considerations of the vascular system** (*Fig. 1-5, A–C*)
   1. **Scimitar syndrome or congenital venolobar syndrome** is lobar hypoplasia or aplasia of the right lung associated with other anomalies of the pulmonary vessels and thorax. Radiographic findings include: small right hemithorax, obscure right heart border, anomalous pulmonary vein that drains into the inferior vena cava and has a Turkish scimitar appearance, and the right pulmonary artery partially absent (replaced by a systemic artery from the aorta).
   2. **Congenital arteriovenous malformation** occurs when there is an abnormal communication between the pulmonary artery and pulmonary vein without an intervening capillary plexus usually found in the lower lobes. Clinical signs include: usually silent in infancy and childhood, but cyanosis, polycythemia, dyspnea, and digital clubbing may be observed.
   3. **Persistent pulmonary hypertension (PPH)** occurs when there is a failure to make the transition from a high pulmonary vascular resistance (PVR) and low blood flow in the fetus to a low PVR and high blood flow in the newborn, most commonly caused by **hypoxia.** If the hypertension causes the ductus arteriosus and foramen ovale to remain open, the condition is called **persistent fetal circulation.** The underlying cause of PPH is smooth muscle thickening of the pulmonary arterioles. Clinical signs include: severe cyanosis, clear lungs, absence of heart disease, decreased pulmonary vascularity, and right-side cardiomegaly.

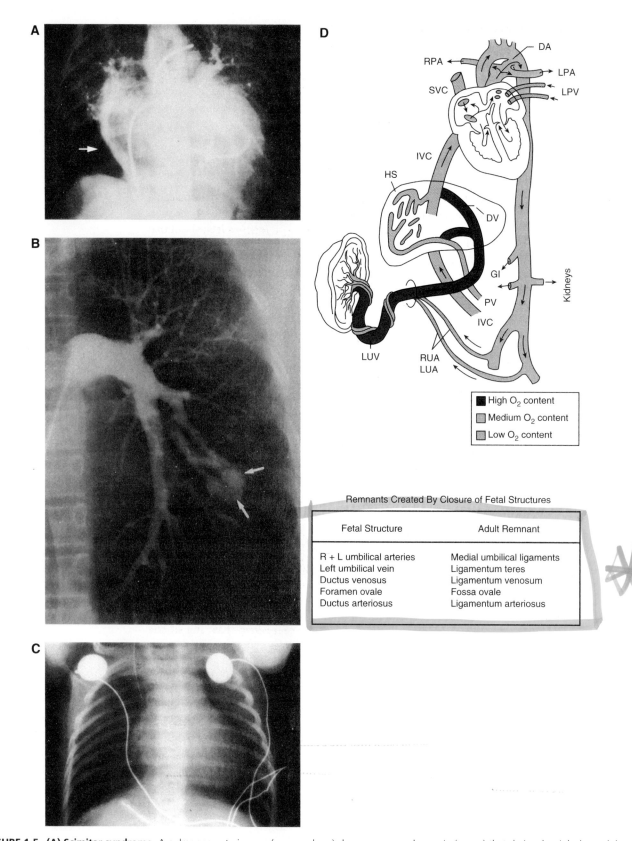

Remnants Created By Closure of Fetal Structures

Fetal Structure	Adult Remnant
R + L umbilical arteries	Medial umbilical ligaments
Left umbilical vein	Ligamentum teres
Ductus venosus	Ligamentum venosum
Foramen ovale	Fossa ovale
Ductus arteriosus	Ligamentum arteriosus

FIGURE 1-5. (A) Scimitar syndrome. A pulmonary arteriogram (venous phase) shows an anomalous vein (*arrow*) that drains the right lower lobe into the inferior vena cava. **(B) Congenital arteriovenous malformation.** A pulmonary angiogram shows a lingular arteriovenous malformation (*arrows*). **(C) Persistent pulmonary hypertension.** AP radiograph shows clear, hypovascularized lungs and an enlarged heart with a right-side pattern. **(D) Diagram of fetal circulation.** RPA—right pulmonary artery; DA—ductus arteriosus; LPA—left pulmonary artery; LPV—left pulmonary veins; SVC—superior vena cava; IVC—inferior vena cava; HS—hepatic sinusoids; DV—ductus venosus; GI—gastrointestinal tract; PV—portal vein; LUV—left umbilical vein; RUA—right umbilical artery; LUA—left umbilical artery.

4. **Anomalous pulmonary venous connection** occurs when none of the four pulmonary veins connects with the left atrium but instead drains into the right atrium, inferior vena cava, or portal vein.

5. **Lobe of the azygos vein** occurs when the right upper lobar bronchus grows medial to the azygos vein, instead of lateral to it. As a result, the azygos vein is found at the bottom of the horizontal fissure of the upper lobe of the right lung. This can be visualized on radiographs as a linear marking.

VII Fetal and Neonatal Circulation (Fig. 1-5D)

A. **Fetal circulation.** The **left umbilical vein** carries high O_2-content blood from the placenta to the **liver,** where 50% of the blood percolates through the **hepatic sinusoids** to the **inferior vena cava (IVC)** and 50% of the blood enters the **ductus venosus** (a fetal shunt that connects the left umbilical vein to the IVC). The **IVC** carries medium O_2-content blood (because the IVC also receives low O_2-content blood from the lower limbs, pelvis, and abdomen via the **portal vein**) to the **right atrium,** where most of the blood enters the **foramen ovale** (a right-to-left fetal shunt that connects the right atrium to the left atrium) and is shunted to the **left atrium,** which also receives low O_2-content blood from the **pulmonary veins.** The **left ventricle** ejects medium O_2-content blood to the **ascending and descending aorta** that perfuses the head/neck and rest of the body, respectively. The remainder of the blood from the IVC and the low O_2-content blood from the **superior vena cava** (SVC) mixes in the right atrium and enters the **right ventricle.** The **right ventricle** ejects medium O_2-content blood to the **pulmonary trunk,** where 10% of the blood enters the lungs and 90% of the blood enters the **ductus arteriosus** (a right-to-left fetal shunt that connects the left pulmonary artery to the arch of the aorta). The **descending aorta** carries medium O_2-content blood, where 35% of the blood is distributed to the fetal body (and returned to the fetal circulation as low O_2-content blood) and 65% of the blood is returned to the placenta by the **right and left umbilical arteries.**

B. **Neonatal circulation.** At birth, the right and left umbilical arteries, left umbilical vein, ductus venosus, ductus arteriosus, and foramen ovale close, cease to function, and form adult remnants. The **right atrial pressure decreases** as a result of occlusion of the placental circulation. The **left atrial pressure increases** as a result of increased pulmonary return from the lungs. The transition from fetal to neonatal circulation is marked when the fluid-filled lungs are distended with air during the first breath. This induces a **rapid decrease in PVR** and an **increased pulmonary blood flow.** The PVR is further reduced by the production of vasodilators, in particular, **prostacyclin** and **nitric oxide** by the neonatal lung. Later, the PVR is further reduced by a **progressive thinning of the smooth muscle layer** (tunica media) of the pulmonary arterial vasculature.

C. **Clinical consideration: patent ductus arteriosus (PDA).** PDA occurs when the ductus arteriosus, a connection between the left pulmonary artery and the arch of the aorta, fails to close. Normally, the ductus arteriosus closes within a few hours after birth via smooth muscle contraction to form the ligamentum arteriosum. PDA causes a **left-to-right shunting** of blood from the aorta back into the pulmonary circulation and is common in **premature infants** and in **maternal rubella** infection. PGE_1, intrauterine asphyxia, and neonatal asphyxia sustain patency of the ductus arteriosus. Prostaglandin inhibitors (e.g., indomethacin), acetylcholine, histamine, and catecholamines promote closure of the ductus arteriosus.

[handwritten margin notes: open: PGE₁, asphyxia; close: PGE inhibs - Indometh, Ach, histamine, catechols]

VIII The Pediatric Thorax (Fig. 1-6)

The chest of a normal newborn infant has a **lampshade or trapezoidal appearance,** which by 6 years of age approaches the long, thin shape seen in the adult. The **posterior mediastinal line,** produced by the right pleuromediastinal reflection, and various **pulmonary fissures** are regularly seen radiographically in newborns and infants.

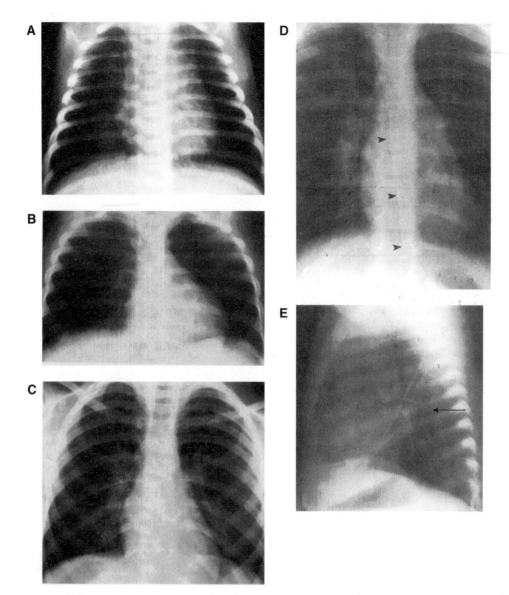

FIGURE 1-6. (A–C) Pediatric thorax. (A) AP radiograph shows a lampshade or trapezoid appearance of the chest in a normal newborn infant. **(B)** AP radiograph of the chest in a 2-year-old normal infant. **(C)** AP radiograph of the chest in a 6-year-old normal child. **(D) Posterior mediastinal line.** AP radiograph shows the posterior mediastinal line (*arrowheads*) in a normal newborn infant. **(E) Oblique fissure.** Lateral radiograph shows the oblique fissure (*arrow*) in a newborn infant.

Chapter 2

Gross Anatomy

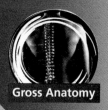

Gross Anatomy

The Thorax

I. Bones of the Thorax

A. **Thoracic vertebrae.** There are 12 thoracic vertebrae that have facets on their bodies (**costal facets**) for articulation with the heads of the ribs, facets on their transverse processes for articulation with the tubercles of the ribs (except for ribs 11 and 12), and long spinous processes.

B. **Ribs.** There are 12 pairs of ribs that articulate with the thoracic vertebrae. A rib consists of **a head, neck, tubercle,** and **body.** The head articulates with the body of adjacent thoracic vertebrae and the intervertebral disc at the **costovertebral joint.** The tubercle articulates with the transverse process of a thoracic vertebra at the **costotransverse joint.**
   1. **True (vertebrosternal) ribs** are **ribs 1–7,** which articulate individually with the sternum by their costal cartilages.
   2. **False (vertebrochondral) ribs** are **ribs 8–12.** Ribs 8–10 articulate with more superior costal cartilage and form the **anterior costal margin.** Ribs 11–12 (often called **floating ribs**) articulate with vertebral bodies but do not articulate with the sternum.

C. The **sternum** consists of the following:
   1. The **manubrium** forms the **jugular notch** at its superior margin, has a **clavicular notch** that articulates with the clavicle at the **sternoclavicular joint,** and articulates with the costal cartilages of ribs 1 and 2.
   2. The **body** articulates with the manubrium at the **sternal angle of Louis,** articulates with the costal cartilages of ribs 2–7, and articulates with the **xiphoid process** at the **xiphosternal joint.**
   3. The **xiphoid process** articulates with the body of the sternum and attaches to the diaphragm and abdominal musculature via the **linea alba.**
   4. The **sternal angle of Louis** marks the junction between the manubrium and body of the sternum at vertebral level T4. This is the site where: ribs 2 articulate with the sternum, the aortic arch begins and ends, the trachea bifurcates, and the superior mediastinum ends.

II. Muscles of the Thorax

A. The **diaphragm (most important muscle of inspiration)** elevates the ribs and increases the vertical, transverse (bucket handle movement), and anteroposterior (pump handle movement) diameters of the thorax. The diaphragm is innervated by the **phrenic nerves** (ventral primary rami of C3–C5), which provide motor and sensory innervation. Sensory innervation to the periphery of the diaphragm is provided by the **intercostal nerves.** A lesion of the phrenic nerve may result in **paralysis** and **paradoxical movement** of the diaphragm. The paralyzed dome of the diaphragm does not

15

descend during inspiration and is consequently forced upward as a result of increased abdominal pressure.

B.   The **intercostal muscles** are thin, multiple layers of muscle that occupy the **intercostal spaces (1–11)** and keep the intercostal space rigid during inspiration or expiration. The **external intercostal muscles** elevate the ribs and play a role in inspiration during exercise or lung disease. The **internal intercostal muscles** play a role in expiration during exercise or lung disease. The **innermost intercostal muscles** are presumed to act with the internal intercostal muscles. The intercostal vein, artery, and nerve run between the internal intercostal muscles and innermost intercostal muscles.

C.   The **sternocleidomastoid, pectoralis major** and **minor,** and the **scalene muscles** attach to the ribs and play a role in inspiration during exercise or lung disease.

D.   The **external oblique, internal oblique, transverse abdominis,** and **rectus abdominis muscles** (i.e., abdominal muscles) play a role in expiration during exercise, lung disease, or the Valsalva maneuver.

 Nerves of the Thorax

The **intercostal nerves** are the ventral primary rami of T1–T11 and run in the **costal groove** between the internal intercostal muscles and innermost intercostal muscles. The **subcostal nerve** is the ventral primary ramus of T12. Intercostal nerve injury is evidenced by a sucking in (upon inspiration) and bulging out (upon expiration) of the affected intercostal space.

 Arteries of the Thorax

A.   The **internal thoracic artery** is a branch of the **subclavian artery** that descends just lateral to the sternum and terminates at intercostal space 6 by dividing into the **superior epigastric artery** and **musculophrenic artery.**

B.   **Anterior intercostal arteries.** The anterior intercostal arteries that supply intercostal spaces 1–6 are branches of the **internal thoracic artery.** The anterior intercostal arteries that supply intercostal spaces 7–9 are branches of the **musculophrenic artery.** There are two anterior intercostal arteries within each intercostal space that anastomose with the posterior intercostal arteries.

C.   **Posterior intercostal arteries.** The posterior intercostal arteries that supply intercostal spaces 1–2 are branches of the **superior intercostal artery** that arises from the **costocervical trunk** of the subclavian artery. The posterior intercostal arteries that supply intercostal spaces 3–11 are branches of the **thoracic aorta.** The **subcostal artery** is also a branch of the thoracic aorta. All posterior intercostal arteries give off a posterior branch that travels with the dorsal primary ramus of a spinal nerve to supply the spinal cord, vertebral column, back muscles, and skin. The posterior intercostal arteries anastomose anteriorly with the anterior intercostal arteries.

 Veins of the Thorax

A.   **Anterior intercostal veins.** The anterior intercostal veins drain the anterior thorax and empty into the **internal thoracic veins,** which then empty into the **brachiocephalic veins.**

B.   **Posterior intercostal veins.** The posterior intercostal veins drain the lateral and posterior thorax and empty into the **hemiazygos veins** on the left side and the **azygos vein** on the right side. The hemiazygos veins empty into the azygos vein, which empties into the superior vena cava.

VI The Breast *(Fig. 2-1)*

A. Components. The breast lies in the superficial fascia of the anterior chest wall over-lying the **pectoralis major** and **serratus anterior muscles** and extends into the **superior lateral quadrant** of the axilla as the **axillary tail,** where a high percentage of tumors occur. In a well-developed female, the breast extends vertically from **rib 2 to rib 6** and laterally from the **sternum to the midaxillary line.** The **retromammary space** lies between the breast and the **pectoral (deep) fascia** and allows free movement of the breast. If breast carcinoma invades the retromammary space and pectoral fascia, contraction of the pectoralis major may cause the **whole breast to move superiorly.** The **suspensory ligaments (Cooper's)** extend from the dermis of the skin to the pectoral fascia and provide support for the breast. If breast carcinoma invades the suspensory ligaments, the ligaments may shorten and cause **dimpling of the skin** or **inversion of the nipple.** The **adipose tissue** within the breast contributes largely to the contour and size of the breast. The **glandular tissue (mammary gland)** within the breast is a modified sweat gland consisting of acini, which are ultimately drained by 15 to 20 **lactiferous ducts** that open onto the nipple. Just deep to the surface of the nipple, each lactiferous duct expands into a **lactiferous sinus,** which serves as a reservoir for milk during lactation. The arterial supply is from the **internal thoracic artery, lateral thoracic artery,** and **intercostal arteries.** The chief venous drainage is to the **axillary vein.** The **internal thoracic, lateral thoracic,** and **intercostal veins** also participate. Metastasis of breast carcinoma to the brain may occur by the following route: cancer cells enter an intercostal vein → external vertebral venous plexuses → internal vertebral venous plexus → cranial dural sinuses. The chief lymphatic drainage is to the **axillary nodes.** Breast carcinoma may metastasize via the lymphatic vessels or block lymph flow, causing a **thick, leathery skin.** The sensory innervation is via **intercostal nerves 2–6 (T2, T3, T4, T5, T6 dermatomes).**

B. Nipple secretion or discharge. Nipple secretion typically contains exfoliated duct cells, α-lactalbumin, immunoglobulins, lactose, cholesterol, steroids, and fatty acids, along with ethanol, caffeine, nicotine, barbiturates, pesticides, and technetium. A nipple discharge that is green, milky, yellow, or brown, not spontaneous, bilateral, and affects multiple ducts is usually a **benign situation.** However, a milky discharge (galactorrhea) along with a headache and peripheral vision loss may indicate a **pituitary adenoma (prolactinoma).** A nipple discharge that is bloody or clear (serous), spontaneous, unilateral, and affects a single duct usually indicates a **malignant situation.**

C. Clinical considerations
1. A **fibroadenoma** is a benign proliferation of connective tissue such that the mammary glands are compressed into cords of epithelium. It presents clinically as a sharply circumscribed, spherical nodule that is freely movable.
2. **Infiltrating duct carcinoma** is a malignant proliferation of duct epithelium in which the tumor cells are arranged in cell nests, cords, anastomosing masses, or a mixture of all these. It is the most common type of breast cancer, accounting for 65 to 80% of all breast cancers. It presents clinically as a jagged density, fixed in position, dimpling of skin, inversion of the nipple, and thick, leathery skin. The presence of the **estrogen receptors** or **progesterone receptors** within the carcinoma cells indicate a good prognosis for treatment. **Tamoxifen** is the drug of choice for treatment of estrogen receptor-positive tumors. The presence of the **c-erb B2 oncoprotein** [a protein similar to the epidermal growth factor (EGF) receptor] on the surface of the carcinoma cells indicates a poor prognosis for treatment. **BRCA 1** (breast cancer susceptibility gene) is an anti-oncogene (tumor suppressor gene) located on chromosome 17 (17q21) that encodes for BRCA protein (a zinc finger gene regulatory protein), containing phosphotyrosine that will suppress the cell cycle. A mutation of the BRCA 1 gene is present in 5 to 10% of women with breast cancer and confers a high lifetime risk of breast and ovarian cancer.

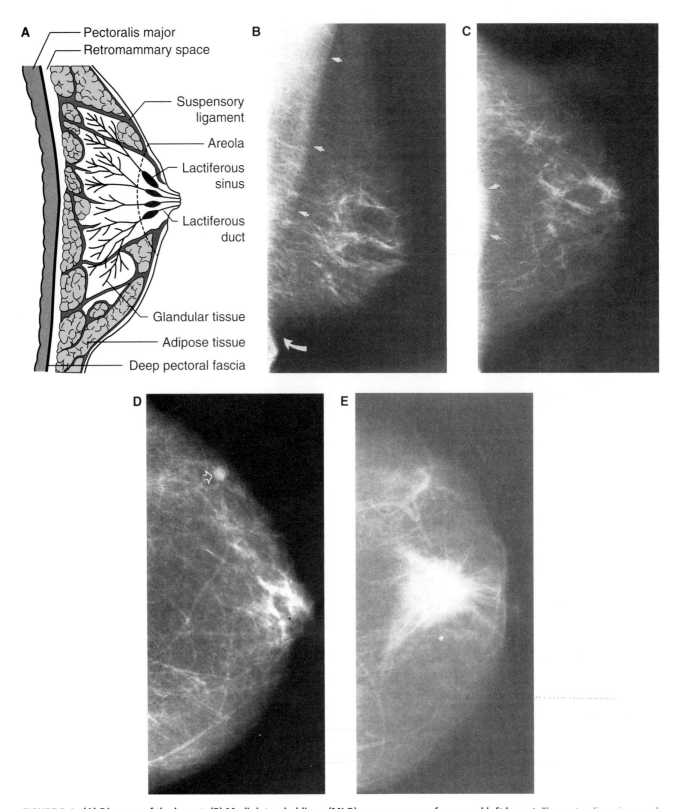

A
Pectoralis major
Retromammary space
Suspensory ligament
Areola
Lactiferous sinus
Lactiferous duct
Glandular tissue
Adipose tissue
Deep pectoral fascia

B

C

D

E

FIGURE 2-1. (A) Diagram of the breast. (B) Mediolateral oblique (MLO) mammogram of a normal left breast. The pectoralis major muscle (*arrows*) and inframammary fold (*curved arrow*) are seen. The nipple is in profile. **(C) Craniocaudal (CC) mammogram of a normal left breast.** The pectoralis major muscle (*arrows*) is seen. **(D) CC mammogram of a benign mass** (*arrow*). A benign mass has the following characteristics: **shape** is round/oval, **margins** are well-circumscribed, **density** is low-medium contrast, becomes smaller over time, and **calcifications** are large, smooth, and uniform. **(E) CC mammogram of a malignant mass.** A malignant mass has the following characteristics: **shape** is irregular with many lobulations, **margins** are irregular or spiculated, **density** is medium to high, breast architecture is distorted, becomes larger over time, and **calcifications** (not shown) are small, irregular, variable, and found within ducts (ductal casts).

3. **Surgical procedures involved in breast cancer**
   a. **Lumpectomy** is the removal of the primary lesion with clear gross margins around the tumor.
   b. **Axillary lymphadenectomy** is the removal of level I lymph nodes (at the lateral border of the pectoralis minor muscle) and level II nodes (behind the pectoralis minor muscle). Level III nodes (at the medial border of the pectoralis minor muscle) are generally not removed.
   c. **Simple mastectomy** removes all breast tissue, including the nipple-areola complex. During a mastectomy, the **long thoracic nerve** must be preserved. Damage to the long thoracic nerve will paralyze the serratus anterior muscle and cause a "winged scapula."
   d. **Modified radical mastectomy (Patey's operation)** removes the skin, entire breast, pectoralis minor muscle, and axillary contents.
   e. **Halsted radical mastectomy** removes the skin, entire breast, pectoralis minor muscle, pectoralis major muscle, and axillary contents.

Ⅶ Clinical Considerations of the Anterior Thorax (*Fig. 2-2*)

A. **Insertion of a central venous catheter.** In clinical practice, access to the superior vena cava (SVC) and right side of the heart is required to monitor blood pressure, long-term feeding, or administration of drugs. The internal jugular vein and subclavian vein are generally used.
   1. **Internal jugular vein (central or anterior approach).** The needle is inserted at the apex of a triangle formed by the two heads of the sternocleidomastoid muscle and the clavicle of the right side.
   2. **Subclavian vein (infraclavicular approach).** Place the index finger at the sternal notch and the thumb at the intersection of the clavicle and first rib as anatomical landmarks. The needle is inserted below the clavicle and lateral to your thumb on the right side.
   3. **Complications of a central venous catheter** may include: puncture of the subclavian artery or subclavian vein, pneumothorax, hemothorax, trauma to the trunks of the brachial plexus, arrhythmias, venous thrombosis, erosion of the catheter through the SVC, damage to the tricuspid valve, and infections.

B. **Postductal coarctation of the aorta** is a congenital malformation associated with increased blood pressure to the upper extremities, diminished and delayed femoral artery pulse, and high risk of cerebral hemorrhage and bacterial endocarditis. A postductal arctation of the aorta is generally located distal to the left subclavian artery and the ligamentum arteriosum. The **internal thoracic artery → intercostal arteries → superior epigastric artery → inferior epigastric artery → external iliac arteries** are involved in the collateral circulation to bypass the constriction and become dilated. The dilation of the intercostal arteries causes erosion of the lower border of the ribs, termed **"rib notching."** A **preductal coarctation** is less common and occurs proximal to the ductus arteriosus; blood reaches the lower part of the body via a patent ductus arteriosus.

C. An **aortic aneurysm** may compress the trachea and tug on the trachea with each cardiac systole such that it can be felt by palpating the trachea at the sternal notch (T2).

D. **Aortic dissection** is defined as a separation of the layers of the aortic wall initiated by either a tear in the weakened tunica intima or rupture of the vasa vasorum with subintimal hemorrhage. Death from aortic dissection is usually from retrograde dissection of blood into the pericardium (causing cardiac tamponade) or into the pleural space.

E. **Thoracic outlet syndrome** may be the result of an anomalous cervical rib and may compress the lower trunk of the brachial plexus and/or subclavian artery. Clinical findings include: atrophy of thenar and hypothenar eminences, atrophy of interosseous muscles,

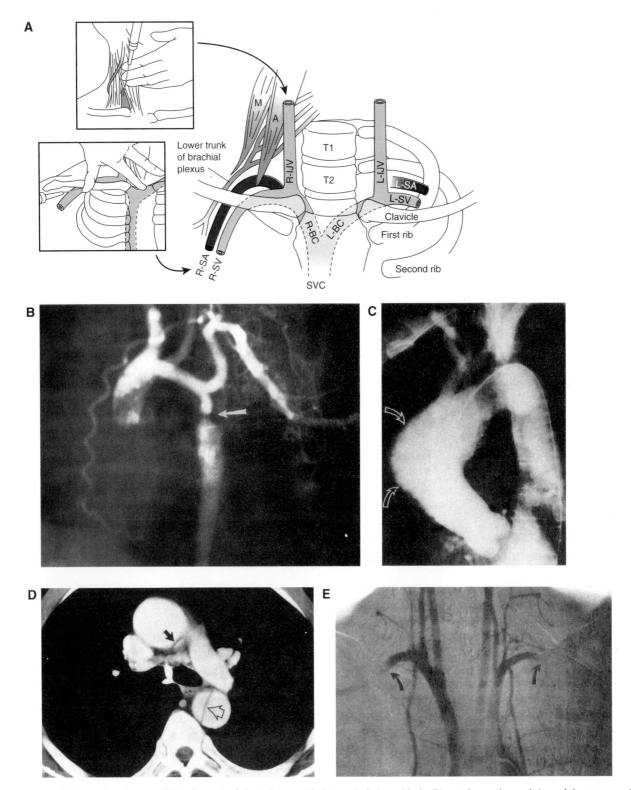

FIGURE 2-2. (A) Anterior chest wall. The first pair of ribs is shown with their articulation with the T1 vertebra and manubrium of the sternum. On the right, structures crossing rib 1 are shown (subclavian vein, subclavian artery, and brachial plexus). Note the relationship of these structures to the clavicle. Note also the arrangement of the large veins in this area and their use in placing a central venous catheter (IJV approach or subclavian approach). L-IJV—left internal jugular vein; L-SV—left subclavian vein; L-BC—left brachiocephalic vein; R-BC—right brachiocephalic vein; SVC—superior vena cava; R-IJV—right internal jugular vein; R-SV—right subclavian vein; R-SA—right subclavian artery. **(B) Postductal coarctation of the aorta.** Angiogram demonstrates a narrowing (*arrow*) just distal to the prominent left subclavian artery. The aortic arch is hypoplastic. Note the tortuous internal thoracic artery. **(C) Aortic aneurysm.** Angiogram shows an atherosclerotic aneurysm (*curved arrows*) protruding from the ascending aorta. **(D) Aortic dissection.** CT scan shows a tunica intima flap within the ascending (*closed arrow*) and descending (*open arrow*) aorta. The larger false lumen compresses the true lumen. **(E) Thoracic outlet syndrome.** Angiogram taken with abduction of both arms shows blood flow is partially occluded in the subclavian arteries (*arrows*).

sensory deficits on the medial side of the forearm and hand, diminished radial artery pulse upon moving the head to the opposite side, and a bruit over the subclavian artery.

F. **Aortic transection** is a result of a deceleration injury (e.g., high-speed motor vehicle accidents) wherein the aorta tears just distal to the left subclavian artery. The tear is in a transverse direction and may involve all three tunics of the aorta.

G. **A knife wound to thorax above the clavicle** may damage the following structures at the root of the neck. The **subclavian artery** may be cut. The **lower trunk of the brachial plexus** may be cut, causing loss of hand movements (ulnar nerve involvement) and loss of sensation over the medial aspect of the arm, forearm, and last two digits (C8 and T1 dermatomes). The **cervical pleura** and **apex of the lung** may be cut, causing an open pneumothorax and collapse of the lung. These structures project superiorly into the neck through the thoracic inlet and posterior to the sternocleidomastoid muscle.

H. **Projections of the diaphragm on the thorax.** The **central tendon of the diaphragm** lies directly posterior to the xiphosternal joint. The **right dome** of the diaphragm arches superiorly to the *upper* border of rib 5 in the midclavicular line. The **left dome** of the diaphragm arches superiorly to the *lower* border of rib 5 in the midclavicular line.

I. **Scalene lymph node biopsy.** Scalene lymph nodes are located behind the clavicle surrounded by pleura, lymph ducts, and the phrenic nerve. Inadvertent damage to the these structures will cause the following clinical findings: pneumothorax, lymph leakage, and diaphragm paralysis, respectively.

Ⅷ Clinical Considerations of the Lateral Thorax *(Fig. 2-3A)*

A. **Intercostal nerve block.** An intercostal nerve block may be necessary to relieve pain associated with a rib fracture or herpes zoster (shingles). A needle is inserted at the posterior angle of the rib along the lower border of the rib to bathe the nerve in anesthetic. The needle penetrates the following structures: **skin → superficial fascia → serratus anterior muscle → external intercostal muscle → internal intercostal muscle.** Several intercostal nerves must be blocked to achieve pain relief because of the presence of nerve collaterals (i.e., overlapping of contiguous dermatomes).

B. **Tube thoracostomy.** Tube thoracostomy is performed to evacuate ongoing production of air/fluid into the pleural cavity. A tube is inserted through intercostal space 5 in the anterior axillary line (i.e., posterior approach) close to the upper border of the rib to avoid the **intercostal vein, artery, and nerve,** which run in the costal groove between the internal intercostal muscle and innermost intercostal muscle. An incision is made at intercostal space 6 lateral to the nipple, but medial to the latissimus dorsi muscle. The tube will penetrate **skin → superficial fascia → serratus anterior muscle → external intercostal muscle → internal intercostal muscle → innermost intercostal muscle → parietal pleura.**

Ⅸ Clinical Considerations of the Posterior Thorax *(Fig. 2-3B)*

A. **Rib fractures.** The **middle ribs** are most commonly fractured just anterior to their **costal angle** (weakest point of the rib). A rib fracture on the right side may damage the **right kidney** and **liver.** A rib fracture on the left side may damage the **left kidney** and **spleen.** A rib fracture on either side may damage the **pleura** as it crosses rib 12. Rib fractures generally are associated with tearing of the intercostal muscles.

B. **Rib dislocation** refers to the displacement of the costal cartilage from the sternum.

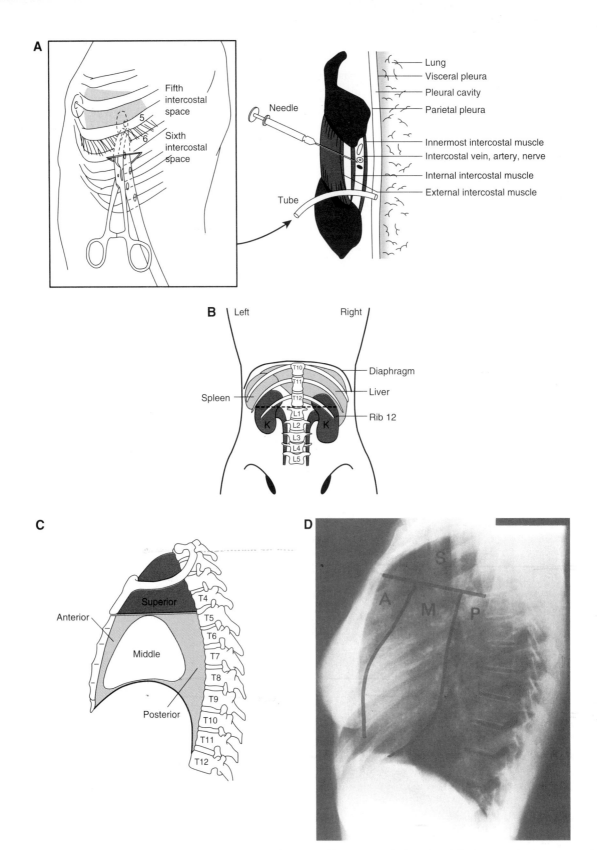

FIGURE 2-3. (A) Lateral chest wall. Diagram shows an intercostal space and layers. Note the location of the intercostal vein, artery, and nerve. Note the relationship of the intercostal space to the pleura and lung. Needle indicates the positioning for an intercostal nerve block. Tube indicates the positioning for a tube thoracostomy. The *inset* demonstrates the surgical approach to inserting a tube for tube thoracostomy. **(B) Posterior chest wall.** Note that the kidneys are located from T12 to L3 vertebrae and that the right kidney is lower than the left. The pleura extends across rib 12 (*dotted line*). Note the structures that may be injured by fractures to the lower ribs. During a splenectomy, the left kidney may be damaged as a result of its close anatomical relationship and connection via the splenorenal ligament. K—kidney. **(C and D) Mediastinum. (C)** Diagram indicating the superior, anterior, middle, and posterior divisions of the mediastinum. **(D)** Lateral radiograph demarcating the superior (*S*), anterior (*A*), middle (*M*), and posterior (*P*) divisions of the mediastinum.

C. **Rib separation** refers to a separation at the costochondral joint (i.e., between the rib and its costal cartilage)

X Mediastinum *(Fig. 2-3, C and D)*

The mediastinum is defined as the space between the pleural cavities in the thorax. It is bounded laterally by the pleural cavities, anteriorly by the sternum, and posteriorly by the vertebral column. The mediastinum is divided into the **superior, anterior, middle,** and **posterior** divisions.

A. **Superior mediastinum.** The contents of the superior mediastinum include the: trachea, esophagus, thymus, phrenic nerves, azygous vein, SVC, brachiocephalic artery and veins, aortic arch, left common carotid artery, left subclavian artery, and thoracic duct. Common pathologies found in this area include: **aortic arch aneurysm, esophageal perforation from either endoscopy or invading malignancy,** or **traumatic rupture of trachea.**

B. **Anterior mediastinum.** The contents of the anterior mediastinum include the: thymus, fat, lymph nodes, and connective tissue. Common pathologies found in this area include: **thymoma associated with myasthenia gravis and RBC aplasia, thyroid mass, germinal cell neoplasm,** or **lymphomas (Hodgkin or non-Hodgkin).**

C. **Middle mediastinum.** The contents of the middle mediastinum include the: heart, pericardium, phrenic nerves, ascending aorta, SVC, IVC (inferior vena cava), and coronary arteries and veins. Common pathologies found in this area include: **pericardial cysts, bronchiogenic cysts,** or **sarcoidosis.**

D. **Posterior mediastinum.** The contents of the posterior mediastinum include the: descending aorta, esophagus, thoracic duct, azygous vein, splanchnic nerves, vagus nerves, and sympathetic trunk. Common pathologies found in this area include: **ganglioneuromas, neuroblastomas,** or **esophageal diverticula or neoplasms.**

Pleura, Tracheobronchial Tree, Lungs

I Pleura

A. **Types of pleura**
1. **Visceral pleura** adheres to the lung on all its surfaces. The visceral pleura is reflected at the root of the lung and continues as parietal pleura.
2. **Parietal pleura** adheres to the chest wall, diaphragm, and pericardial sac. The parietal pleura is named according to the anatomical region it is associated with.
    a. **Costal pleura** is associated with the internal surface of the sternum, costal cartilages, ribs, and sides of the thoracic vertebrae.
    b. **Mediastinal pleura** is associated with the mediastinum and forms the **pulmonary ligament** (located inferior to the root of the lung), which serves to support the lung.
    c. **Diaphragmatic pleura** is associated with the diaphragm.
    d. **Cervical pleura** is associated with the root of the neck.

B. **Pleural recesses**
1. **Right and left costodiaphragmatic recesses** are slitlike spaces between the costal and diaphragmatic parietal pleura. During inspiration, the lungs descend into the right and left costodiaphragmatic recesses, causing the recesses to appear radiolucent

(dark) on radiographs. During expiration, the lungs ascend so that the costal and diaphragmatic parietal pleura come together and the radiolucency disappears on radiographs. The costodiaphragmatic angle should appear sharp in a PA radiograph. If the angle is blunted, pathology of the pleural space may be suspected, such as excess fluid, blood, tumor, or scar tissue. With a patient in the standing position, excess fluid within the pleural cavity will accumulate in the costodiaphragmatic recesses.

2. **Right and left costomediastinal recesses** are slitlike spaces between the costal and mediastinal parietal pleura. During inspiration, the anterior borders of both lungs expand and enter the right and left costomediastinal recesses. In addition, the **lingula of the left lung** expands and enters a portion of the *left* costomediastinal recess, causing that portion of the recess to appear radiolucent (dark) on radiographs. During expiration, the anterior borders of both lungs recede and exit the right and left costomediastinal recesses.

C. **Clinical considerations**
1. **Pleuritis** is inflammation of the pleura. Pleuritis involving only visceral pleura will be associated with **no pain** because the visceral pleura receives no nerve fibers of general sensation. Pleuritis involving the parietal pleura will be associated with **sharp local pain** and **referred pain.** Because parietal pleura is innervated by intercostal nerves and the phrenic nerve (C3, C4, C5), pain may be referred to the **thoracic wall** and **root of the neck,** respectively.
2. **Inadvertent damage to the pleura** may occur during a(n):
   a. **Surgical posterior approach to the kidney.** If rib 12 is very short, rib 11 may be mistaken for rib 12. An incision prolonged to the level of rib 11 will damage the pleura.
   b. **Abdominal incision at the right infrasternal angle.** The pleura extends beyond the rib cage in this area.
   c. **Stellate ganglion nerve block**
   d. **Brachial plexus nerve block**
   e. **Knife wounds to the chest wall above the clavicle**
   f. **Fracture of lower ribs**
3. A **chylothorax** occurs when lymph accumulates in the pleural cavity as a result of surgery or trauma that injures the thoracic duct.
4. **Spontaneous pneumothorax** (*Fig. 2-4A*) occurs when air enters the pleural cavity, usually as a result of a ruptured bleb (bullous) of a diseased lung. The most common site is in the visceral pleura of the upper lobe of the lung. This results in a loss of negative intrapleural pressure and a **collapsed lung.** Clinical findings include: chest pain, cough, and mild to severe dyspnea.
5. **Open pneumothorax** occurs when the parietal pleura is pierced and the pleural cavity is opened to the outside atmosphere. This causes a loss of the negative intrapleural pressure (P_{IP}) because P_{IP} now equals atmospheric pressure (P_{atm}). This results in an expanded chest wall (its natural tendency) and a collapsed lung (its natural tendency). Upon inspiration, air is sucked into the pleural cavity and results in a **collapsed lung.** Most common causes include: chest trauma (e.g., knife wound) and iatrogenic etiology (e.g., thoracocentesis, transthoracic lung biopsy, mechanical ventilation, or central line insertion).
6. **Tension pneumothorax** (Fig. 2-4B) may occur as a sequela to an open pneumothorax if the inspired air cannot leave the pleural cavity through the wound upon expiration (check valve mechanism). This results in a **collapsed lung** on the wounded side and a **compressed lung** on the opposite side as a result of a deflected mediastinum. Clinical findings include: chest pain, shortness of breath, absent breath sounds on the affected side, and hypotension because the mediastinal shift compresses the SVC and IVC, thereby obstructing venous return. May cause sudden death.

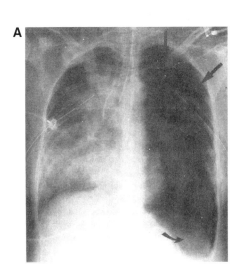
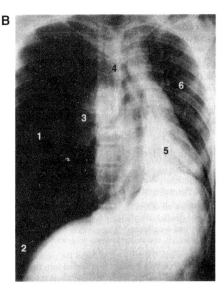

FIGURE 2-4. (A) Pneumothorax. PA radiograph shows a left apical (*arrows*) and subpulmonic (*curved arrow*) pneumothorax in a 41-year-old woman with ARDS. **(B) Tension pneumothorax.** AP radiograph shows a tension pneumothorax as a result of a penetrating chest trauma to the right side. 1—hyperlucent lung field; 2—hyperexpansion lowers right diaphragm; 3—collapsed right lung; 4—deviation of trachea; 5—mediastinal shift; 6—compressed left lung.

⓾ Tracheobronchial Tree (*Fig. 2-5A*)

A. General characteristics. The trachea is a tube composed of **16 to 20 U-shaped hyaline cartilages** and the **trachealis** muscle. The trachea begins just inferior to the cricoid cartilage (C6 vertebral level) and ends at the sternal angle (T4 vertebral level), where it bifurcates into the **right and left main bronchi.**

At the bifurcation of the trachea, the last tracheal cartilage forms the **carina**, which can be observed by bronchoscopy as a raised ridge of tissue in the sagittal plane. The right main bronchus is shorter, wider, and turns to the right at a shallower angle than the left main bronchus. The right main bronchus branches into **3 lobar bronchi** (upper, middle, and lower) and finally into **10 segmental bronchi.** The left main bronchus branches into **2 lobar bronchi** (upper and lower) and finally into **8–10 segmental bronchi.** The branching of segmental bronchi corresponds to the **bronchopulmonary segments** of the lung.

B. Clinical considerations

1. **Compression of the trachea** may be caused by **enlargement of the thyroid gland** or an **aortic arch aneurysm.** The aortic arch aneurysm may tug on the trachea with each cardiac systole such that it can be felt by palpating the trachea at the sternal notch.

2. **Distortions in the position of the carina** may indicate **metastasis of bronchogenic carcinoma** into the tracheobronchial lymph nodes that surround the tracheal bifurcation or may indicate **enlargement of the left atrium.** The mucous membrane covering the carina is very sensitive in eliciting the cough reflex.

3. **Aspiration of foreign objects.**
   a. **When a person is sitting or standing.** Aspirated material most commonly enters the **right lower lobar bronchus** and lodges within the **posterior basal bronchopulmonary segment (#10) of the right lower lobe.**

   post lower – sit/stand

   b. **When a person is supine.** Aspirated material most commonly enters the **right lower lobar bronchus** and lodges within the **superior bronchopulmonary segment (#6) of the right lower lobe.**

   sup lower – supine

   c. **When a person is lying on the right side.** Aspirated material most commonly enters the **right upper lobar bronchus** and lodges within the **posterior bronchopulmonary segment (#2) of the right upper lobe.**

   post upper – lying R side
   inf upper – lying L side

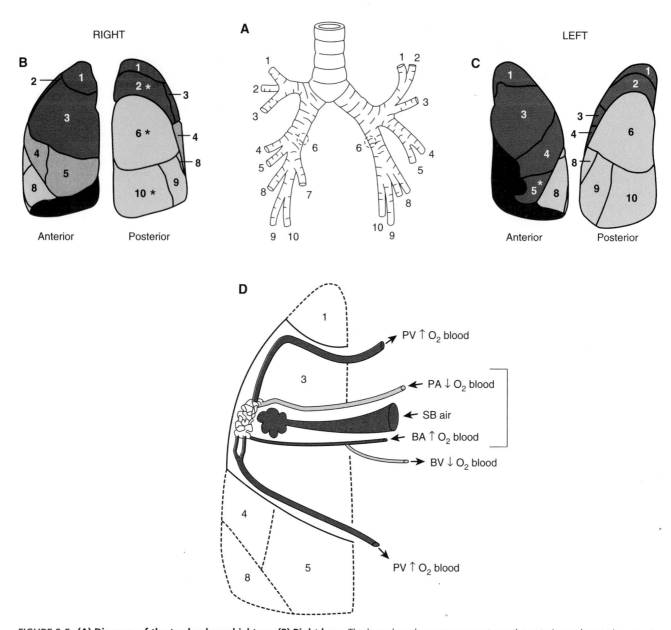

FIGURE 2-5. (A) Diagram of the tracheobronchial tree. (B) Right lung. The bronchopulmonary segments on the anterior and posterior aspects of the right lung are indicated. 1—apical; 2—posterior; 3—anterior; 4—lateral; 5—medial, 6—superior; 8—anterior basal; 9—lateral basal; 10—posterior basal. Note that #7 (medial basal) is located on the inner mediastinal surface (not shown)., **(C) Left lung.** The bronchopulmonary segments on the anterior and posterior aspects of the left lung are indicated. 1—apical; 2—posterior; 3—anterior; 4—superior lingular; 5—inferior lingular; 6—superior; 8—anterior basal; 9—lateral basal; 10—posterior basal. Note there is no #7 segmental bronchus or bronchopulmonary segment in the left lung. *—the bronchopulmonary segments involved in aspiration of foreign objects. **(D) Bronchopulmonary segment.** Diagram of bronchopulmonary segment #3 of the right lung shows the centrally located segmental bronchus #3 (*SB*), branch of the pulmonary artery (*PA*), and branch of the bronchial artery (*BA*). Note the location of the pulmonary veins (*PV*) at the periphery of the bronchopulmonary segment. Bronchial veins (*BV*) are also indicated. 1, 4, 5, and 8—bronchopulmonary segments.

   d. **When a person is lying on the left side.** Aspirated material most commonly enters the **left upper lobar bronchus** and lodges within the **inferior lingular (#5) bronchopulmonary segment of the left upper lobe.**

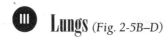 **Lungs** (Fig. 2-5B–D)

A. **The right lung** consists of **three lobes (upper, middle, and lower)** separated by a **horizontal fissure** and an **oblique fissure.** The right upper lobe lies in a superior/anterior position. The right middle lobe lies in an anterior position between costal cartilages 4 and 6. The right lower lobe lies in an inferior/posterior position. The horizontal fissure runs at the level of costal cartilage 4 and meets the oblique fissure at the midaxillary line. The **diaphragmatic surface** consists of the middle lobe and lower lobe.

B. The **left lung** consists of **two lobes (upper and lower)** separated by an **oblique fissure.** The left upper lobe lies in a superior/anterior position and contains the **cardiac notch** where the left ventricle and pericardial sac abut the lung. The **lingula** (which is the embryological counterpart to the right middle lobe) lies just beneath the cardiac notch. The left lower lobe lies in an inferior/posterior position. The **diaphragmatic surface** consists of the lower lobe.

C. A **bronchopulmonary segment** contains a **segmental bronchus**, a **branch of the pulmonary artery,** and a **branch of the bronchial artery,** which run together through the **central** part of the segment. It contains **tributaries of the pulmonary vein,** which are found at the **periphery** between two adjacent bronchopulmonary segments. These veins form surgical landmarks during segmental resection of the lung. The bronchopulmonary segments are both named and numbered as indicated below:
1. **Right lung**
   a. **Upper lobe:** apical (#1), **posterior (#2)***, anterior (#3)
   b. **Middle lobe:** lateral (#4), medial (#5)
   c. **Lower lobe: superior (#6),** medial basal (#7), anterior basal (#8), lateral basal (#9), **posterior basal (#10)**
2. **Left lung**
   a. **Upper lobe:** apical (#1), posterior (#2), anterior (#3), superior lingular (#4), **inferior lingular (#5)**
   b. **Lower lobe:** superior (#6), anterior basal (#8), lateral basal (#9), posterior basal (#10). Note #7 is absent.
      * Bronchopulmonary segments in bold are most frequently involved in aspiration of foreign objects.

D. **Breath sounds**
1. Breath sounds from the upper lobe of each lung can be auscultated on the anterior–superior aspect of the thorax.
2. Breath sounds from the lower lobe of each lung can be auscultated on the posterior–inferior aspect of the back.
3. Breath sounds from the middle lobe of the right lung can be auscultated on the anterior thorax near the sternum just inferior to intercostal space 4.

E. **Vasculature of the lung.** The adult lung is supplied by two arterial systems and drained by two venous systems.
1. The **pulmonary trunk** is anterior to the ascending aorta and travels in a superior–posterior direction to the left side for about 5 cm and then bifurcates into the **right pulmonary artery** and **left pulmonary artery,** which carry deoxygenated blood to the lung for aeration. The **right pulmonary artery** runs horizontally towards the hilus beneath the arch of the aorta, posterior to the ascending aorta and superior vena cava, and anterior to the right main bronchus. The **left pulmonary artery** is shorter and narrower than the right pulmonary artery and is connected to the arch of the aorta by the **ligamentum arteriosum.** The pulmonary arteries branch to follow the airways to the level of the terminal bronchiole, at which point they form a pulmonary capillary plexus.
2. The **bronchial arteries** carry oxygenated blood to the parenchyma of the lung. The **right bronchial artery** is a branch of a posterior intercostal artery. The two **left bronchial arteries** are branches of the thoracic aorta. The bronchial arteries branch to follow the airways to the level of the terminal bronchioles at which point they drain into the **pulmonary capillary plexus** (i.e., 70% of bronchial blood drains into

the pulmonary capillary plexus). Bronchial arteries that supply large bronchi drain into **bronchial veins** (i.e., 30% of bronchial blood drains into the bronchial veins).

3. The **pulmonary veins** carry oxygenated blood from the pulmonary capillary plexus and deoxygenated bronchial blood to the left atrium. There are five pulmonary veins that drain each lobe of the lungs. However, the pulmonary veins from the right upper and middle lobes generally join so that only **four pulmonary veins** open into the posterior aspect of the **left atrium.** Within the lung, small branches of the pulmonary veins run **solo** (i.e., do not run with the airways, pulmonary arteries, or bronchial arteries). Larger branches of the pulmonary veins are found at the periphery of the bronchopulmonary segments (i.e., **intersegmental location**).

4. The **bronchial veins** carry deoxygenated blood from the bronchial arteries that supply large bronchi. **<u>Right bronchial veins</u> drain into the <u>azygos vein</u>. Left bronchial veins drain into the accessory hemiazygos vein.**

F. Innervation of the lung (*Fig. 2-6A*). The lungs are innervated by the **anterior pulmonary plexus** and **posterior pulmonary plexus,** which are located anterior and posterior to the root of the lung at the hilus, respectively. These plexuses contain both **parasympathetic (vagus; CN X)** and **sympathetic components.**

1. Parasympathetic. Preganglionic neuronal cell bodies are located in the **dorsal nucleus of the vagus** and **nucleus ambiguus** of the medulla. Preganglionic axons run in the **vagus nerve (CN X).** Postganglionic neuronal cell bodies are located in the **pulmonary plexuses** and **within the lung** along the bronchial airways. Postganglionic parasympathetic axons terminate on the smooth muscle of the bronchial tree, causing **bronchoconstriction,** and seromucous glands, causing **increased glandular secretion.** Postganglionic parasympathetic axons release **acetylcholine (ACh)** as a neurotransmitter, which binds to muscarinic ACh receptors (a G protein-linked receptor). Afferent (sensory) nerve fibers run with CN X and carry touch and stretch modalities.

2. Sympathetic. Preganglionic neuronal cell bodies are located in the **intermediolateral cell column** of the spinal cord. Preganglionic axons enter the **paravertebral ganglion.** Postganglionic neuronal cells bodies are located in the paravertebral ganglion at the cervical (superior, middle, and inferior ganglia) and thoracic (T1–T4) levels. Postganglionic sympathetic axons terminate on postganglionic parasympathetic neurons and modulate their bronchoconstriction activity (thereby causing **bronchodilation**). Circulating epinephrine from the adrenal medulla acts directly on bronchial smooth muscle to cause bronchodilation. Postganglionic sympathetic axons also terminate on the smooth muscle of blood vessels, causing **vasoconstriction.** Postganglionic sympathetic axons release **norepinephrine (NE)** as a neurotransmitter, which binds to adrenergic receptors (a G protein-linked receptor).

G. Lymphatic drainage of the lung (Fig. 2-6B). The adult lung has lymphatic plexuses that communicate freely. Lymph from the right lung ultimately drains into the **right bronchomediastinal trunk,** which empties into the junction of the right internal jugular vein and right subclavian vein. Most of the lymph from the left lung ultimately drains into the **left bronchomediastinal trunk,** which empties into the junction of the left internal jugular vein and left subclavian vein. Lymph from the lower lobe of the left lung drains into the right lung pathway.

1. The **superficial plexus** of lymphatic vessels lie just deep to the visceral pleura and drain lymph to the **bronchopulmonary lymph nodes** → **inferior and superior tracheobronchial lymph nodes** → **paratracheal lymph nodes** → **bronchomediastinal trunk.**

2. The **deep plexus** of lymphatic vessels lie in the submucosa and connective of bronchi and drain lymph to **pulmonary lymph nodes** → **bronchopulmonary lymph nodes** → **inferior and superior tracheobronchial lymph nodes** → **paratracheal lymph nodes** → **bronchomediastinal trunk.**

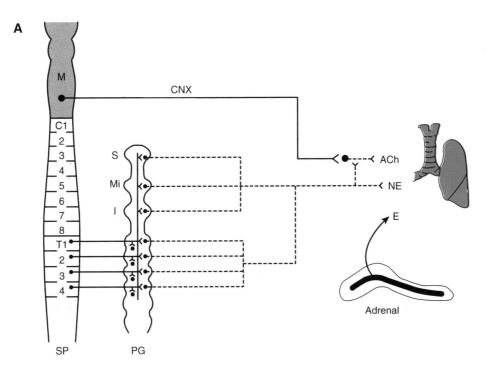

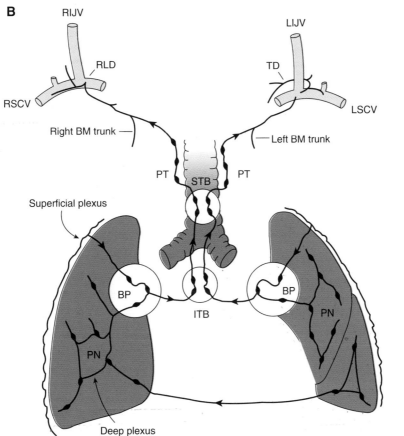

FIGURE 2-6. (A) Innervation of the lung. Parasympathetic innervation involving the vagus nerve (CN X) is shown. Sympathetic innervation is also shown. The adrenal medulla secretes epinephrine (*E*), which causes bronchodilation. All preganglionic neurons are indicated by *solid lines*. All post-ganglionic neurons are indicated by *dotted lines*. M—medulla; SP—spinal cord; PG—paravertebral ganglia; S—superior cervical ganglia; Mi—middle cervical ganglia; I—inferior cervical ganglia; ACh—acetylcholine; NE—norepinephrine. **(B) Lymphatic drainage of the lung.** Diagram indicates the pattern of the superficial plexus and deep plexus of the lung. PN—pulmonary nodes; BP—bronchopulmonary nodes; ITB—inferior tracheo-bronchial nodes; STB—superior tracheobronchial nodes; PT—paratracheal nodes; BM—bronchomediastinal; TD—thoracic duct; RLD—right lymphatic duct; RSCV—right subclavian vein; LSCV—left subclavian vein; RIJV—right internal jugular vein; LIJV—left internal jugular vein.

Chapter 3

Radiology

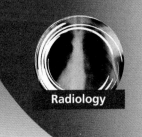
Radiology

I Posterior-Anterior (PA) Chest Film

The film cassette is placed against the chest and the x-ray beam is directed at the back and travels in a posterior-anterior direction (hence the name). The routine PA chest film is taken with the patient upright and in full inspiration. A normal chest film shows four densities listed from less radiodense (black) → more radiodense (white): the air density of the lungs; fat density around the muscles; water density of the heart, muscle, and blood; and bone density of the ribs and vertebrae.

II Anterior-Posterior (AP) Chest Film

The film cassette is placed against the back and the x-ray beam is directed at the chest and travels in an anterior-posterior direction (hence the name). The AP chest film is usually performed on very sick patients, who are unable to stand, and infants. The patient is usually supine or sitting up in bed.

III Lateral Chest Film

The film cassette is placed against left side of the chest and the x-ray is directed at the right side of the chest and travels from the right side to the left side.

IV Lung Fissures

Knowing the location of lung lobes on chest films is critical for understanding patterns of lung disease and clinical diagnosis. If the x-ray beam is parallel to a fissure, the fissure will be visible on the radiograph. If the x-ray beam is oblique to a fissure, the fissure will not be visible on the radiograph.

A. **Right lung:** The oblique fissure is visible only on a lateral chest film. The horizontal fissure is visible on both the PA and lateral chest films.

B. **Left lung:** The oblique fissure is visible only on a lateral chest film.

V Bronchopulmonary Segments

Each lobe of the lung is further subdivided into bronchopulmonary segments based on the distribution of segmental bronchi. Knowing the location of lung lobes on chest films is critical for understanding patterns of lung disease and clinical diagnosis.

VI Signs

A. **Air bronchogram sign** refers to a branching, linear, or tubular radiolucency that represents a bronchus or bronchiole passing through an airless portion of the lung parenchyma.

B. **Air crescent sign** refers to a peripheral crescent-shaped radiolucency that occurs when a portion of the lung undergoes necrosis and cavitation. The radiolucency is located between the wall of the cavity and the mass within the cavity.

C. **Continuous diaphragm sign** refers to a continuous radiolucency outlining the base of the heart, indicating a pneumomediastinum in which air in the mediastinum tracks outside the pleura between the heart and diaphragm.

D. **CT angiogram sign** refers to the presence of prominent blood vessels within an airless portion of the lung parenchyma on a contrast-enhanced CT scan.

E. **Deep sulcus sign** refers to a collection of air within the pleural cavity (i.e., a pneumothorax) located in the costophrenic recess.

F. **Fallen lung sign** refers to a collapsed lung that results from a fractured bronchus. The lung "falls" away from the hilum in an inferior-lateral direction. In contrast, a collapsed lung caused by a pneumothorax collapses in a medial direction toward the hilum.

G. **Flat waist sign** refers to the flattening of the aortic knob and pulmonary trunk on the left border of the cardiovascular shadow that results from a severe collapse of the lower lobe of the left lung.

H. **Gloved finger sign** refers to bronchi that are impacted with mucus, cellular debris, and fungal hyphae, generally as a result of allergic bronchopulmonary aspergillosis.

I. **Golden S sign** refers to the reverse S-shape of a fissure involved when a lobe collapses around a large, central mass (e.g., bronchogenic carcinoma). In this situation, the peripheral portion of the lobe collapses but the central portion of the lobe does not collapse, because of the presence of the mass. This distorts the normally straight-shaped fissure into a reverse S-shape.

J. **Halo sign** refers to a ground-glass halo that forms around a lung consolidation seen in a CT scan and is highly suggestive of invasive pulmonary aspergillosis.

K. **Hampton hump sign** refers to a rounded hump of abnormal radiodensity in contact with the pleural surface, as a result of a pulmonary infarction secondary to a pulmonary embolism.

L. **Juxtaphrenic peak sign** refers to a small, triangular shadow that obscures the dome of the right hemidiaphragm as a result of atelectasis of the upper lobe of the right lung.

M. **Luft Sichel sign** refers to a sickle-shaped radiolucency around the aortic knob resulting from hyperinflation of the superior bronchopulmonary segment of the lower lobe of the left lung that occurs when the upper lobe of the left lung collapses. This sign indicates the probable diagnosis of bronchogenic carcinoma.

N. **Melting ice cube sign** refers to a melting (in a peripheral → internal direction) ice cube appearance of a resolving pulmonary infarction.

O. **Ring around the artery sign** refers to a ring-shaped radiolucency around the right pulmonary artery (seen on a lateral chest film) as a result of a pneumomediastinum.

P. **Silhouette sign** refers to the obliteration of the borders of the heart, other mediastinal structures, or diaphragm as a result of an adjacent radiodensity. A radiodensity in the medial bronchopulmonary segment of the middle lobe of the right lung obliterates the right heart border. A radiodensity in the lingula of the left lung obliterates the left heart border. A radiodensity in the basal bronchopulmonary segments of the right or left lung obliterates the border of the diaphragm.

Q. **Split pleura sign** refers to the splitting of the thickened visceral and parietal pleura into two separate structures on a CT scan as a result of fluid accumulation from empyema. Normally, the visceral and parietal pleura cannot be distinguished as two separate structures.

R. Westermark sign refers to the decreased amount of circulating blood (oligemia) in the lung beyond the point of blood vessel occlusion as a result of a pulmonary embolism.

Ⅶ Selected Radiographs, CT, and MRI

A. PA chest radiograph *(Fig. 3-1)*

B. Lateral chest radiograph *(Fig. 3-2)*

C. Lung fissures *(Fig. 3-3)*

D. Bronchopulmonary segments *(Figs. 3-4 and 3-5)*

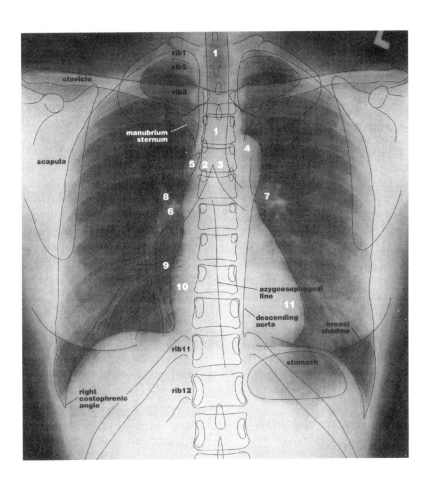

1: Trachea	7: Left pulmonary artery
2: Right main bronchus	8: Right upper lobe pulmonary artery
3: Left main bronchus	9: Right inferior pulmonary vein
4: Aortic knob	10: Right atrium
5: Azygos vein/SVC	11: Left ventricle
6: Right pulmonary artery	

FIGURE 3-1. PA chest radiograph. Note the various numbered and labeled structures. Ribs 1–8 generally can be traced from their articulation with the vertebral column to the union of the rib with the costal cartilage. The liver and right dome of the diaphragm cast a domed water-density shadowed at the base of the right lung. The stomach, spleen, and left dome of the diaphragm cast a domed water-density shadowed at the base of the left lung. Both domes generally lie just below vertebra T10. The left dome is lower than the right dome because of the downward thrust of the heart. The right border of the cardiovascular shadow includes the: brachiocephalic artery and right brachiocephalic vein, superior vena cava and ascending aorta, right atrium, and inferior vena cava. The left border of the cardiovascular shadow includes the: left subclavian artery and left brachiocephalic vein, aortic arch (or aortic knob), pulmonary trunk, auricle of left atrium, and left ventricle. The angle between the right and left main bronchi at the carina is generally 60–75°. The left hilum is generally higher than the right hilum.

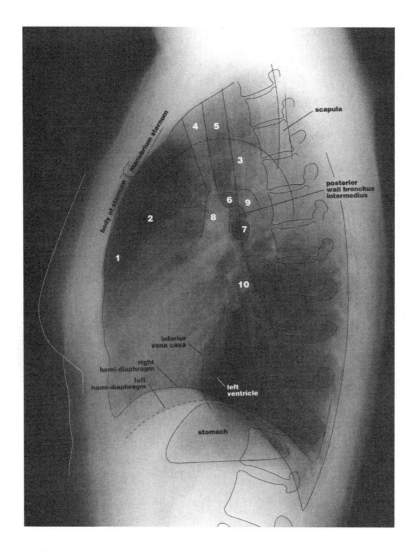

1: Pulmonary outflow tract
2: Ascending aorta
3: Aortic arch
4: Brachiocephalic vessels
5: Trachea

6: Right upper lobar bronchus
7: Left upper lobar bronchus
8: Right pulmonary artery
9: Left pulmonary artery
10: Confluence of pulmonary veins

FIGURE 3-2. Lateral chest radiograph. Note the various numbered and labeled structures.

E. **CT scan at the level of origin of the three branches of the aortic arch (about vertebral level T2–T3)** *(Fig. 3-6)*

F. **CT scan and MRI at the level of the aortic arch** *(Fig. 3-7)*

G. **CT scan (*A*) and MRI (*B*) at the level of the aortic-pulmonary window (at about vertebral level T4)** *(Fig. 3-8)*

H. **CT scan at the level of the origin of the left pulmonary artery** *(Fig. 3-9)*

I. **CT scan (*A*) and MRI (*B*) at the level of the origin of the right pulmonary artery (at about vertebral level T6)** *(Fig. 3-10)*

J. **CT scan (*A*) and MRI (*B*) at the level of the origin of the ascending aorta and pulmonary trunk at the right ventricle (at about vertebral level T6)** *(Fig. 3-11)*.

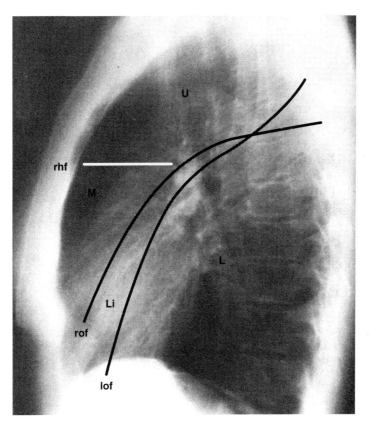

FIGURE 3-3. Lung fissures. A lateral chest film shows the orientation of the right horizontal fissure (*rhf*), right oblique fissure (*rof*), and left oblique fissure (*lof*). The right oblique fissure and left oblique can be distinguished from each other by the following characteristics: 1) the right horizontal fissure ends on the right oblique fissure, 2) the left oblique fissure ends on the left diaphragm, which usually has a stomach gas bubble immediately beneath it. After identifying the fissures, one can accurately locate the lobes of the lung as indicated by the letters. U—upper lobes of the lungs; L—lower lobes of the lung; M—right middle lobe; Li—lingula.

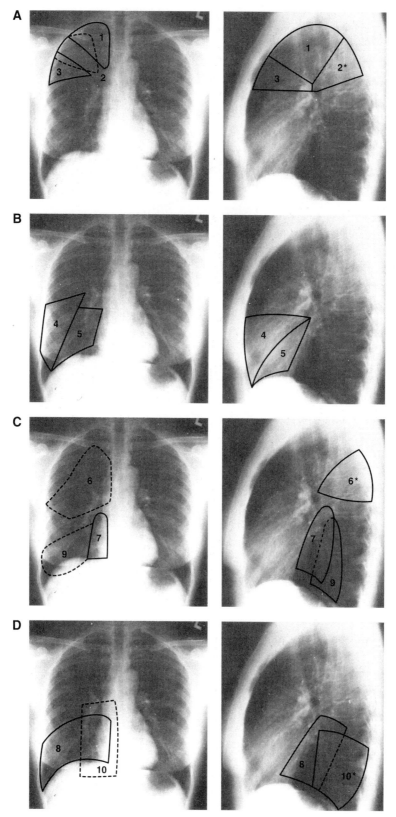

FIGURE 3-4. Right lung bronchopulmonary segments. (A) PA and lateral chest films show the orientation of the apical (*1*), posterior (*2*), and anterior (*3*) bronchopulmonary segments of the upper lobe of the right lung. **(B)** PA and lateral chest films show the orientation of the lateral (*4*) and medial (*5*) bronchopulmonary segments of the middle lobe of the right lung. **(C)** PA and lateral chest films show the orientation of the superior (*6*), medial basal (*7*), and lateral basal (*9*) bronchopulmonary segments of the lower lobe of the right lung. **(D)** PA and lateral chest films show the orientation of the anterior basal (*8*) and posterior basal (*10*) bronchopulmonary segments of the lower lobe of the right lung. *—bronchopulmonary segments involved in aspiration of foreign objects.

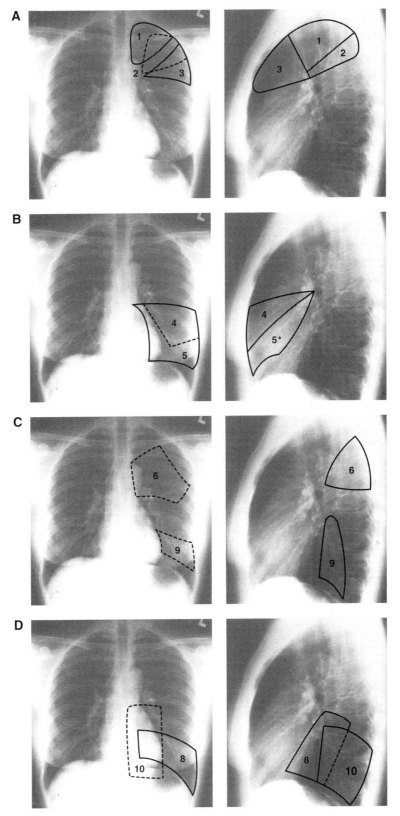

FIGURE 3-5. Left lung bronchopulmonary segments. (A) PA and lateral chest films show the orientation of the apical (*1*), posterior (*2*), and anterior (*3*) bronchopulmonary segments of the upper lobe of the left lung. **(B)** PA and lateral chest films show the orientation of the superior lingular (*4*) and inferior lingular (*5*) bronchopulmonary segments of the upper lobe of the left lung. **(C)** PA and lateral chest films show the orientation of the superior (*6*) and lateral basal (*9*) bronchopulmonary segments of the lower lobe of the left lung. Note that the medial basal (*7*) bronchopulmonary segment is absent in the left lung. **(D)** PA and lateral chest films show the orientation of the anterior basal (*8*) and posterior basal (*10*) bronchopulmonary segments of the lower lobe of the left lung. *—bronchopulmonary segment involved in aspiration of foreign objects.

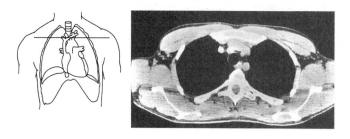

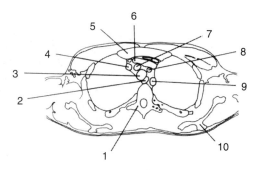

1. Thoracic vertebra
2. Esophagus
3. Trachea
4. Rt. brachiocephalic vein
5. Sternum

6. Lt. brachiocephalic vein
7. Brachiocephalic trunk
8. Lt. common carotid artery
9. Lt. subclavian vein
10. Scapula

FIGURE 3-6. CT scan at the level of origin of the three branches of the aortic arch (about vertebral level T2–T3). The esophagus is anterior and to the left of the body of the thoracic vertebra. The trachea is anterior and to the right of the esophagus. The brachiocephalic trunk is anterior and to the right of the trachea. The left common carotid artery is anterior and to the left of the trachea. The left subclavian artery is to the left of the posterior border of the trachea. The right brachiocephalic vein is to the right of the brachiocephalic trunk. The left brachiocephalic vein appears in oblique section as it travels to the right side.

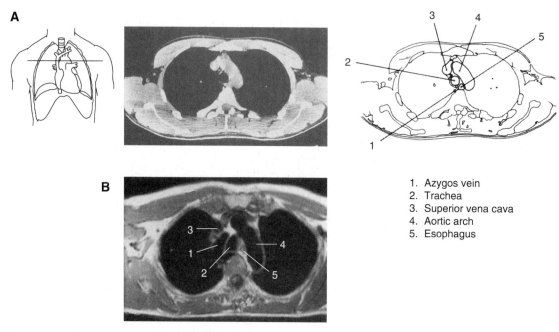

1. Azygos vein
2. Trachea
3. Superior vena cava
4. Aortic arch
5. Esophagus

FIGURE 3-7. CT scan (A) and MRI (B) at the level of the aortic arch. The esophagus is anterior and to the left of the body of the thoracic vertebra. The trachea is anterior and to the right of the esophagus. The azygos vein is posterior to the trachea and to the right of the esophagus. The aortic arch is a curved image that begins to the left of the superior vena cava (or right brachiocephalic vein), curves around the trachea, and ends to the left of the esophagus. The left brachiocephalic vein appears in oblique section at its union with the right brachiocephalic vein emptying into the superior vena cava.

A

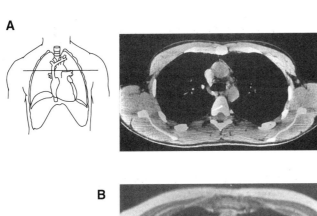

B

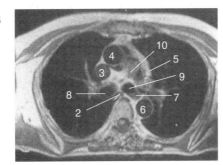

1. Trachea
2. Azygos vein
3. Superior vena cava
4. Ascending aorta
5. Aortic-pulmonary window

6. Descending aorta
7. Esophagus
8. Rt. main bronchus
9. Lt. main bronchus
10. Pulmonary trunk

FIGURE 3-8. CT scan (A) and MRI (B) at the level of the aortic-pulmonary window (at about vertebral level T4). The aortic-pulmonary window is the space in the superior mediastinum from the bifurcation of the pulmonary trunk to the undersurface of the aortic arch. The esophagus is anterior and to the left of the body of the thoracic vertebra. At this level, the trachea bifurcates into the right main bronchus and left main bronchus. The azygos vein appears in longitudinal section as it arches over the right main bronchus and empties into the superior vena cava. The ascending aorta is anterior to the right main bronchus; and, anterior and to the left of the superior vena cava.

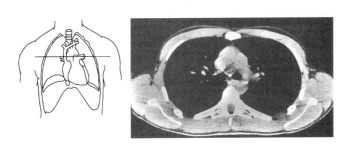

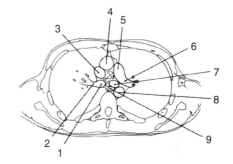

1. Rt. main bronchus
2. Branching of rt. main bronchus
3. Superior vena cava
4. Ascending aorta

5. Pulmonary trunk
6. Lt. pulmonary artery
7. Lt. main bronchus
8. Descending aorta
9. Esophagus

FIGURE 3-9. CT scan at the level of the origin of the left pulmonary artery. The left main bronchus appears in cross-section anterior to the esophagus and descending aorta. The right main bronchus branches into the right upper lobar bronchus and right middle lobar bronchus. The pulmonary trunk is anterior and to the left of the left main bronchus. The left pulmonary artery appears in longitudinal section as it curves posterior-lateral towards the hilum of the left lung. The superior vena cava is anterior to the right main bronchus. The ascending aorta is anterior and between the right main bronchus and left main bronchus.

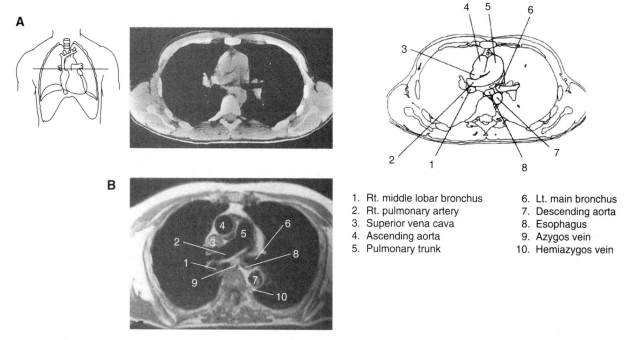

1. Rt. middle lobar bronchus
2. Rt. pulmonary artery
3. Superior vena cava
4. Ascending aorta
5. Pulmonary trunk
6. Lt. main bronchus
7. Descending aorta
8. Esophagus
9. Azygos vein
10. Hemiazygos vein

FIGURE 3-10. CT scan (A) and MRI (B) at the level of the origin of the right pulmonary artery (at about vertebral level T5). At this level, the left main bronchus bifurcates into the upper lobar bronchus and lower lobar bronchus. The pulmonary trunk is anterior to the left main bronchus. The right pulmonary artery appears in longitudinal section as it curves posterior to the ascending aorta and superior vena cava and anterior to the right middle lobar bronchus as it travels toward the hilum of the right lung.

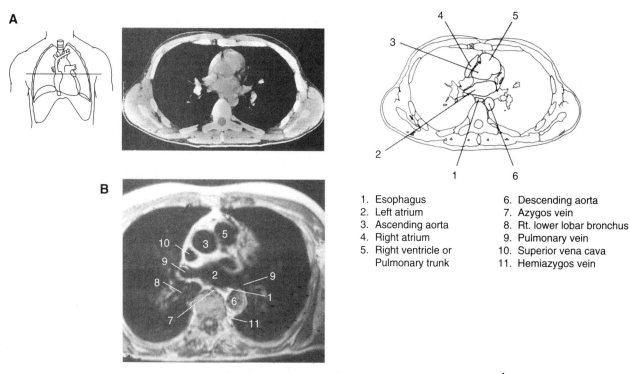

1. Esophagus
2. Left atrium
3. Ascending aorta
4. Right atrium
5. Right ventricle or Pulmonary trunk
6. Descending aorta
7. Azygos vein
8. Rt. lower lobar bronchus
9. Pulmonary vein
10. Superior vena cava
11. Hemiazygos vein

FIGURE 3-11. CT scan (A) and MRI (B) at the level of the origin of the ascending aorta and pulmonary trunk at the right ventricle (at about vertebral level T6). The origins of the ascending aorta and pulmonary trunk lie anterior to the left atrium. The crescent-shaped right atrium lies to the right of the ascending aorta.

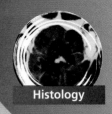
Chapter 4

Histology

I General Features (Fig. 4-1)

The respiratory system is divided into a **conduction portion** and a **respiratory portion.** The conduction portion **only conducts air into the lung;** no blood–air gas exchange occurs. Airflow through the conduction portion follows this route: **nasal cavities → nasopharynx → oropharynx → larynx → trachea → bronchi → bronchioles → terminal bronchioles.** The respiratory portion is where **blood–air gas exchange occurs.** Airflow through the respiratory portion follows this route: **respiratory bronchioles → alveolar ducts → alveoli.** The larger airways of the conduction portion (i.e., trachea and bronchi) are organized into a **mucosa (epithelium and lamina propria), muscular layer, submucosa,** and **adventitia.** As the airways get progressively smaller down to the alveoli, the components of the wall change significantly and this organization is lost.

II Trachea

A. **Mucosa.** The epithelium is a **respiratory epithelium,** which is classically described as a **ciliated pseudostratified epithelium with goblet cells** that contain the following cell types. **Ciliated cells** (≅30%) beat toward the pharynx, thereby moving mucus and/or particulate matter to the mouth where it can be swallowed or expectorated. **Goblet cells** (≅30%) secrete mucous. **Brush cells** contain microvilli and have been interpreted as either an intermediate stage in the differentiation to ciliated cells or as a sensory cell, since they may be found in association with nerve terminals. **Endocrine cells (Kulchitsky cells)** secrete peptide hormones and catecholamines. **Basal cells** (≅30%) have mitotic capacity and thereby function as stem cells to regenerate the epithelium. The lamina propria consists of **collagen and elastic fibers.**

B. **Muscular layer.** The muscular layer consists of smooth muscle that spans the dorsal ends of the cartilage rings, called the **trachealis muscle.**

C. **Submucosa.** The submucosa consists of **seromucous glands** surrounded by **collagen and elastic fibers.**

D. **Adventitia.** The adventitia consists of **C-shaped hyaline cartilage rings** surrounded by **collagen and elastic fibers.**

III Bronchi

A. **Mucosa.** The epithelium is a **respiratory epithelium** as described above. The lamina propria consists of **collagen and elastic fibers.**

B. **Muscular layer.** The muscular layer consists of a **prominent circular layer of smooth muscle.**

C. **Submucosa.** The submucosa consists of **seromucous glands** surrounded by **collagen and elastic fibers.**

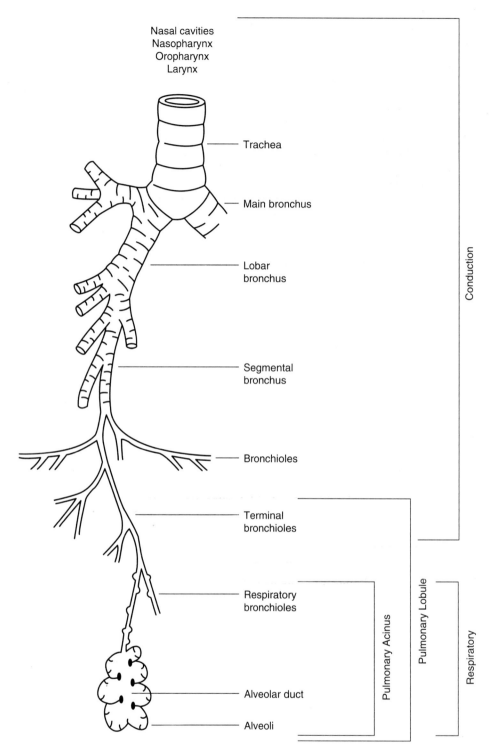

Nasal cavities
Nasopharynx
Oropharynx
Larynx

Trachea

Main bronchus

Lobar
bronchus

Segmental
bronchus

Bronchioles

Terminal
bronchioles

Respiratory
bronchioles

Alveolar duct

Alveoli

Conduction

Pulmonary Acinus

Pulmonary Lobule

Respiratory

FIGURE 4-1. Diagram of the respiratory system. The conduction portion of the respiratory system begins with the nasal cavities and ends with the terminal bronchioles (hence their name). The respiratory portion of the respiratory system begins with the respiratory bronchioles (hence their name) and ends with the alveoli. A pulmonary lobule consists of a terminal bronchiole, respiratory bronchioles, alveolar ducts, and alveoli. A pulmonary acinus consists of a respiratory bronchiole, alveolar duct, and alveoli. Note that respiratory bronchioles are distinguished histologically by the presence of alveoli that open into their wall. The pulmonary lobule–pulmonary acinus concept is important pathologically in classifying types of emphysema: 1) centriacinar emphysema involves widening of air spaces within the respiratory bronchioles only at the apex of an acinus, whereas 2) panacinar emphysema involves widening of air spaces distal to the terminal bronchiole involving the entire acinus.

D. **Adventitia.** The adventitia consists of **irregular hyaline cartilage plates** surrounded by **collagen and elastic fibers.**

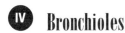 Bronchioles

A. **Mucosa.** The epithelium is a **simple ciliated columnar epithelium** with **goblet cells** and **Clara cells.** The lamina propria consists of **collagen and elastic fibers.** Clara cells **secrete a component of surfactant, secrete Clara cell protein (CC16),** which is used as a marker of pulmonary function in bronchopulmonary lavage fluid and serum, **metabolize airborne toxins** using cytochrome P-450, and **release Cl⁻** into the lumen via a Cl⁻ ion channel regulated by a cGMP-guanylate cyclase mechanism. Clara cells are nonciliated, have a dome-shaped protrusion extending into the lumen, and have the ultrastructural characteristics of a protein-secreting cell (rER, Golgi, secretory granules).

B. **Muscular layer.** The muscular layer consists of a **prominent circular layer of smooth muscle.**

Terminal Bronchioles

A. **Mucosa.** The epithelium is a **simple ciliated cuboidal epithelium** with **Clara cells.** The lamina propria consists of **collagen and elastic fibers.**

B. **Muscular layer.** The muscular layer consists of a **reduced, incomplete circular layer of smooth muscle.**

Respiratory Bronchioles

A. **Mucosa.** The epithelium is a **simple ciliated cuboidal epithelium** with numerous **Clara cells.** The lamina propria consists of **collagen and elastic fibers.**

B. **Muscular layer.** The muscular layer consists of a **prominent, incomplete circular layer of smooth muscle.** Note that respiratory bronchioles are distinguished histologically by the presence of alveoli that open into its wall.

Alveolar Ducts

A. **Mucosa.** The epithelium is a **simple squamous epithelium.** The lamina propria consists of **collagen and elastic fibers.**

B. **Muscular layer.** The muscular layer consists of **smooth muscle "knobs."**

Alveoli

Alveoli contain the following:

A. **Type I pneumocytes** are a simple squamous epithelium joined by tight junctions (zonula occludens) that line alveoli and have no mitotic capacity.

B. **Type II pneumocytes** are cuboidal-shaped cells that are most commonly found at the junction of interalveolar septae and bulge into the air space. These cells secrete **surfactant** (which is stored as **lamellar bodies**) and have mitotic capacity, thereby functioning as stem cells to regenerate the epithelium. Hyperplasia of type II pneumocytes is an important marker of alveolar injury and repair of alveoli.

C. Alveolar macrophages migrate over the surface of the alveoli and into the interalveolar septae to phagocytose inhaled dust, bacteria, and degraded surfactant.

D. Alveolar pores (pores of Kohn) are found within interalveolar septae and equalize pressure within alveoli. These pores play a significant role in obstructive lung disease by serving as a bypass to aerate alveoli distal to the blockage. The **interalveolar septae** of the alveoli contain **collagen and elastic fibers.**

Ⅸ Surfactant

Surfactant is composed of **cholesterol (50%), dipalmitoylphosphatidylcholine (DPPC; 40%), and surfactant proteins (10%) SP-A, SP-B, and SP-C.** SP-A and SP-B combine with DPPC in the lamellar bodies within type II pneumocytes. SP-B and SP-C stabilize the surfactant coat. Surfactant lines the alveoli and reduces surface tension, which prevents the collapse of small alveoli (atelectasis), cyanosis, and respiratory distress. Surfactant is the major contributor to the **elastance** of the lung. **Elastance** is the collapsing force that develops in the lung as the lung expands and is described by the **Laplace law** (see Physiology section).

Ⅹ Blood-Air Barrier

The components of the blood-air barrier include the: **surfactant layer, type I pneumocyte, basement membrane,** and **capillary endothelial cell.** The rate of diffusion across the blood-air barrier is governed by the **Fick law** (see Physiology section). Note that increases in the thickness of the blood-air barrier will decrease the rate of diffusion of O_2 and CO_2 across the blood-air barrier.

Ⅺ Air Flow

Airflow through the lung from the bronchi to alveoli is inversely proportional to **airway resistance** and is described by the **Poiseuille law** (see Physiology section). The **medium-sized bronchi** are the **main site of airway resistance** through the contraction or relaxation of smooth muscle.

A. Parasympathetic stimulation, leukotrienes (LTC$_4$, LTD$_4$), PGF$_{2\alpha}$, and thromboxane (TXA$_2$) constrict the airways (i.e., reduce the radius) and thereby increase airway resistance. These are called **bronchoconstrictors.**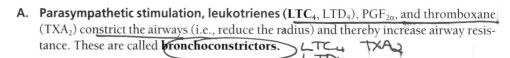

B. Sympathetic stimulation, PGE$_2$, and β$_2$-adrenergic agonists (e.g., Terbutaline, Albuterol, Metaproterenol, Salmeterol) dilate the airways (i.e., increase the radius) and thereby decrease airway resistance. These are called **bronchodilators.**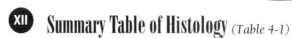

Ⅻ Summary Table of Histology *(Table 4-1)*

TABLE 4-1		SUMMARY TABLE OF HISTOLOGY		
	Mucosa	**Smooth Muscular Layer**	**Submucosa**	**Adventitia**
Trachea	Respiratory epithelium	Trachealis muscle	Seromucous glands	C-shaped hyaline cartilage rings
	Collagen and elastic fibers		Collagen and elastic fibers	Collagen and elastic fibers
Bronchi	Respiratory epithelium	Prominent circular layer	Seromucous glands	Irregular hyaline cartilage plates
	Collagen and elastic fibers		Collagen and elastic fibers	Collagen and elastic fibers
Bronchioles	Simple ciliated columnar with Goblet cells and Clara cells Collagen and elastic fibers	Prominent circular layer	Absent	Absent
Terminal bronchioles	Simple ciliated cuboidal with Clara cells Collagen and elastic fibers	Reduced, incomplete circular layer	Absent	Absent
Respiratory bronchioles	Simple ciliated cuboidal with Clara cells Collagen and elastic fibers	Prominent, incomplete circular layer	Absent	Absent
Alveolar ducts	Simple squamous epithelium Collagen and elastic fibers	Smooth muscle "knobs"	Absent	Absent
Alveoli	Type I pneumocytes Type II pneumocytes Alveolar macrophages Collagen and elastic fibers	Absent	Absent	Absent

XIII Selected Photomicrographs

A. Trachea, bronchus, bronchiole, and pulmonary lobule (Fig. 4-2)

B. Clara cells, type II pneumocytes, and alveolar macrophages (Fig. 4-3)

C. Alveoli, interalveolar wall, and blood-air barrier (Fig. 4-4)

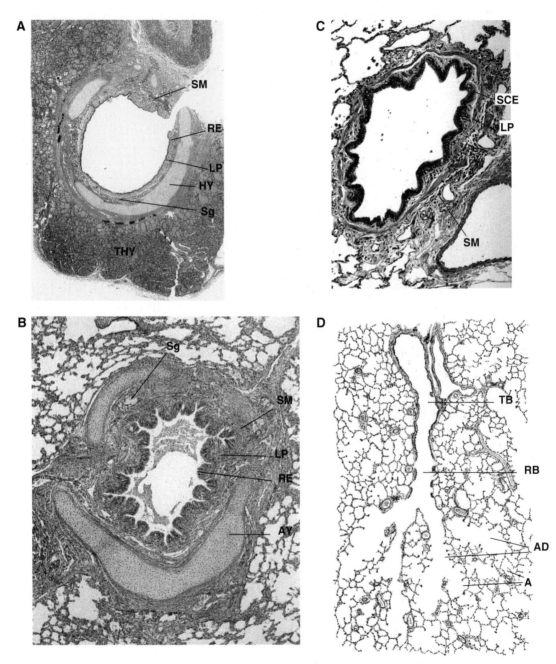

FIGURE 4-2. **(A) LM of the trachea.** This LM shows a low magnification cross-section through the entire trachea. Note the respiratory epithelium (RE) lining the lumen with the underlying lamina propria (LP) containing collagen and elastic fibers. The smooth muscle (SM) trachealis muscle is shown at the dorsal ends of the hyaline cartilage (HY). Seromucous glands (Sg) are located in the submucosa. A portion of the thyroid gland (THY) is also shown. **(B) LM of a bronchus.** Note the respiratory epithelium (RE), lamina propria (LP), smooth muscle (SM), seromucous glands (Sg), and irregular hyaline cartilage plates (HY). **(C) LM of a bronchiole.** Note the simple ciliated columnar epithelium (SCE), lamina propria (LP), and smooth muscle (SM). **(D) LM of a pulmonary lobule.** Note that the terminal bronchiole (TB) is continuous with a respiratory bronchiole (RB), which then branches into alveolar ducts (AD). The alveolar ducts open into the alveoli (A). Note that respiratory bronchioles are distinguished histologically by the presence of alveoli that open into its wall.

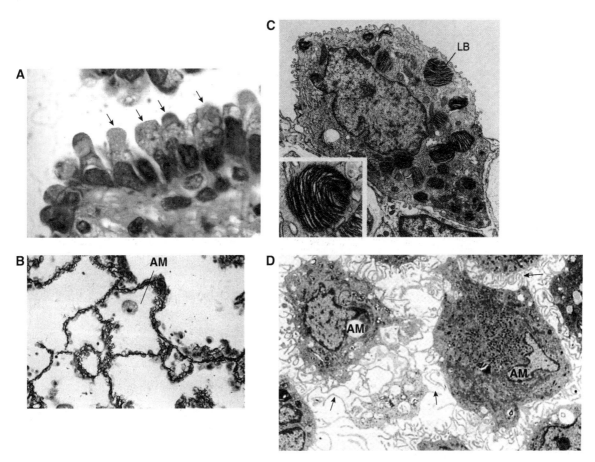

FIGURE 4-3. (A) LM of Clara cells. Note that Clara cells (*arrows*) are nonciliated and have a dome-shaped protrusion extending into the lumen. Clara cells are found in both terminal bronchioles and respiratory bronchioles. **(B) EM of a type II pneumocyte.** Type II pneumocytes contain lamellar bodies (*LB*), which contain surfactant. The high magnification inset shows the unique appearance of a lamellar body. **(C) LM of an alveolar macrophage.** Note the alveolar macrophage (*AM*) in the alveolar lumen. **(D) EM of alveolar macrophages.** These alveolar macrophages were isolated from an individual exposed to silica. Note the activation of the alveolar macrophages as evidenced by the numerous filopodia (*arrows*) extending from the cell surface.

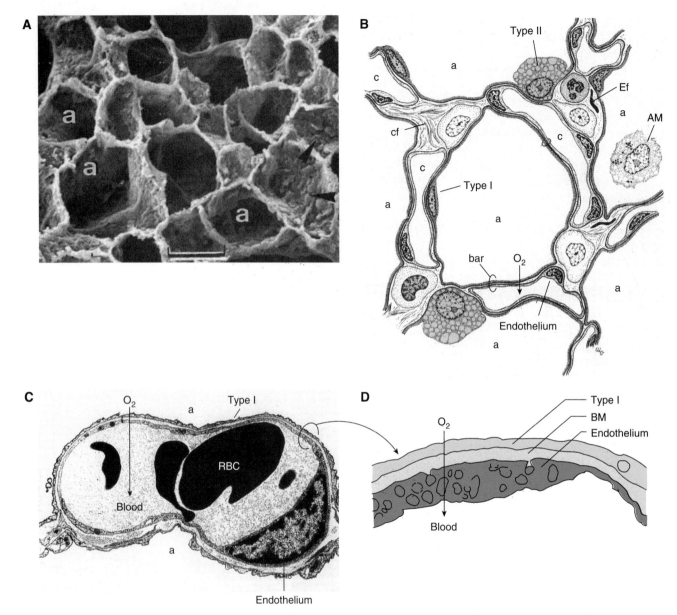

FIGURE 4-4. (A) SEM of alveoli. This SEM shows numerous alveoli (*a*). Note that the wall of the alveoli (i.e., the interalveolar wall) is corrugated or rough (*arrows*) because of the presence of capillaries within the interalveolar wall bulging into the alveolar lumen. **(B) Diagram of the interalveolar wall.** Note the alveolar lumen (*a*) where air of O_2 is present and the capillaries (*c*) where blood is present. Type I pneumocytes are shown lining the alveoli and capillary endothelium is shown lining the capillaries. The type I pneumocytes and capillary endothelium along with the basement membrane make up the blood-air barrier (*bar*). Type II pneumocytes and alveolar macrophages (*AM*) are shown. The presence of collagen fibers (*Cf*) and elastic fibers (*Ef*) are shown within the interalveolar septae. **(C) EM of a capillary within the interalveolar wall.** A cross-section of a capillary lined by endothelium (*Endo*) and containing red blood cells (*RBC*) is shown. This capillary is bordered on both sides by alveoli (*a*) containing air or O_2 and lined by type I pneumocytes. Note the route of diffusion of O_2 from the alveolar lumen to the blood. **(D) EM of the blood-air barrier.** This high-magnification EM clearly shows the components of the blood-air barrier, namely the type I pneumocytes, basement membrane (*BM*), and capillary endothelium. Note the route of diffusion of O_2 from the alveolar lumen to the blood must cross these components. The surfactant layer is not visible.

Chapter 5

Physiology

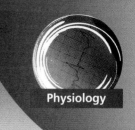

Lung Mechanics

I ## Lung Volumes and Capacities *(Fig. 5-1)*

A. **Static pulmonary mechanics** refers to the mechanical forces acting on the lung and chest wall that determine lung volume. **Lung volumes** are compartments of the lung that contain air and are measured by various techniques (lung volumes are not visible on radiographs). **Lung capacities** are two or more volumes that are added together. The lung increases in size from birth to late teens, plateaus, then declines with aging. Age-related changes in the lung volumes include: decrease in vital capacity (VC), total lung capacity (TLC), and expiratory reserve volume (ERV); increase in residual volume (RV); no change in functional residual capacity (FRC).

B. **The physiologic role of FRC.** Breathing is a cyclical process whereas blood flow through the lung capillary bed is a continuous process. During the respiratory cycle, short periods of apnea occur at which time there is no ventilation but blood flow continues. The FRC acts as a reservoir for continued gas exchange during the apneic periods. Without FRC, high levels of deoxygenated blood from the pulmonary capillaries would empty into pulmonary veins and consequently lower the partial pressure of arterial oxygen (P_{aO2}). This would in effect constitute an intrapulmonary shunt.

II ## Breathing

A. **Muscles involved in breathing**
1. **Inspiration.** During normal breathing, the **diaphragm** is the most important muscle in inspiration. Contraction of the diaphragm elevates the ribs, which causes an anterior expansion (pump handle movement) and lateral expansion (bucket handle movement) of the thorax. During exercise or lung disease, the **external intercostal, sternocleidomastoid, pectoralis major** and **minor,** and **scalene muscles** play a role in inspiration.
2. **Expiration.** During normal breathing, expiration is a **passive process** because the chest wall-lung unit is elastic and recoils to its resting position after inspiration. During exercise or lung disease, the **internal intercostal muscles, external oblique, internal oblique, transversus abdominus, and rectus abdominus muscles** play a role in expiration. Maximal expiratory pressure is reached by fully contracting the expiratory muscles with the lungs completely inflated against a closed glottis (i.e., the **Valsalva maneuver**). The Valsalva maneuver is commonly performed when lifting a heavy object or during defecation.

B. **The breathing cycle** *(Fig. 5-2).* In order to understand the breathing cycle, three parameters are considered:
1. **Lung volumes,** particularly the **functional residual capacity (FRC)** and **tidal volume (TV).**
2. **Alveolar pressure (P_A)** is expressed relative to atmospheric pressure (P_{atm}; 760 mm Hg at sea level). When P_A equals P_{atm}, the P_A is said to be **zero.** When P_A is greater

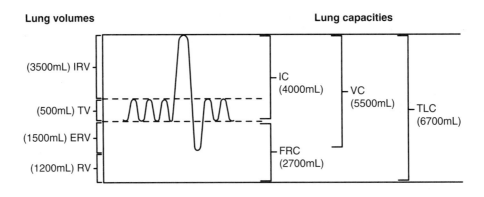

Volume/Capacity	Normal Value	Description
Inspiratory Reserve Volume (IRV)	3500mL	Volume inspired above the tidal volume
Tidal Volume (TV)	500mL	Volume of a normal breath
Expiratory Reserve Volume (ERV)	1500mL	Volume expired after expiration of tidal volume Decreases with age
Residual Volume (RV)	1200mL	Volume that remains after maximal expiration Increases with age Cannot be measured by spirometry RV = FRC − ERV
Inspiratory Capacity (IC)	4000mL	IC = IRV + TV
Functional Residual Capacity (FRC)	2700mL	Volume remaining after TV is expired No change with age FRC = ERV − RV
Vital Capacity (VC)	5500mL	Volume expired after maximal inspiration Decreases with age VC = TLC − RV
Total Lung Capacity (TLC)	6700mL	Volume that lung can maximally hold Decreases with age TLC = IRV + TV + ERV + RV
Dead Space (DS)	Anatomic DS = 150mL	**Anatomic DS:** Portion of the breath that remains in the conducting airways **Alveolar DS:** Portion of the breath entering alveoli that receive no or reduced blood flow **Physiologic DS:** Portion of breath that does not participate in gas exchange **Physiologic DS = Anatomic DS + Alveolar DS**
Forced Vital Capacity (FVC)	5500mL	Volume forcibly expired after maximal inspiration Pulmonary function tests measure FVC
Forced Expiratory Volume (FEV$_1$)	4400mL (80% of FVC) FEV$_1$/FVC=0.8	Volume expired in 1 second during an FVC maneuver

* Physiologic DS = TV x $\dfrac{P_{aco_2} - P_{Eco_2}}{P_{aco_2}}$ where TV = tidal volume, P_{aco_2} = P_{co_2} of arterial blood, P_{Eco_2} = P_{co_2} of expired air

FIGURE 5-1. Spirometry diagram of lung volumes and capacities.

A

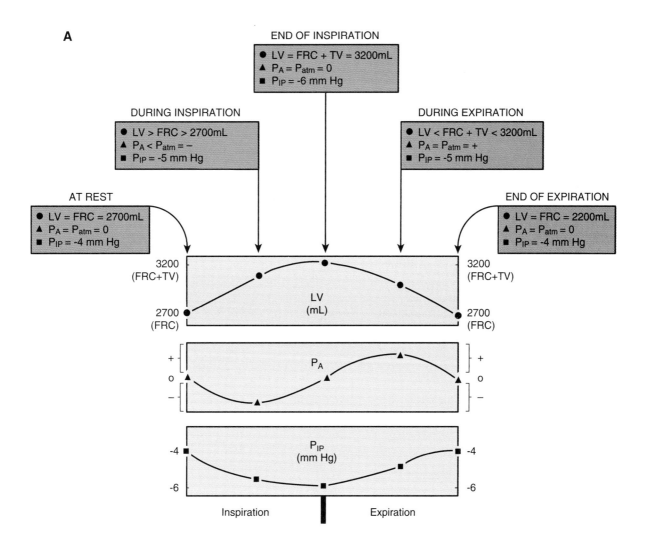

END OF INSPIRATION
- ● LV = FRC + TV = 3200mL
- ▲ P_A = P_{atm} = 0
- ■ P_{IP} = -6 mm Hg

DURING INSPIRATION
- ● LV > FRC > 2700mL
- ▲ P_A < P_{atm} = −
- ■ P_{IP} = -5 mm Hg

DURING EXPIRATION
- ● LV < FRC + TV < 3200mL
- ▲ P_A = P_{atm} = +
- ■ P_{IP} = -5 mm Hg

AT REST
- ● LV = FRC = 2700mL
- ▲ P_A = P_{atm} = 0
- ■ P_{IP} = -4 mm Hg

END OF EXPIRATION
- ● LV = FRC = 2200mL
- ▲ P_A = P_{atm} = 0
- ■ P_{IP} = -4 mm Hg

3200 (FRC+TV)   3200 (FRC+TV)
2700 (FRC)   2700 (FRC)
LV (mL)

P_A
+ 0 −   + 0 −

P_{IP} (mm Hg)
-4   -4
-6   -6

Inspiration   Expiration

B

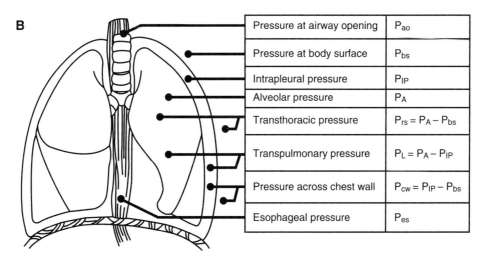

Pressure at airway opening	P_{ao}
Pressure at body surface	P_{bs}
Intrapleural pressure	P_{IP}
Alveolar pressure	P_A
Transthoracic pressure	$P_{rs} = P_A − P_{bs}$
Transpulmonary pressure	$P_L = P_A − P_{IP}$
Pressure across chest wall	$P_{cw} = P_{IP} − P_{bs}$
Esophageal pressure	P_{es}

FIGURE 5-2. (A) Breathing cycle. Diagram of the breathing cycle showing the changes in lung volume, alveolar pressure, and intrapleural pressure. When discussing the breathing cycle, pressures are generally expressed in centimeters of water (cm H_2O) because small pressures are involved. So that at rest, the P_{IP} = −5 cm H_2O. A pressure of 1 cm H_2O = 0.74 mm Hg. So that, −5 × 0.74 mm Hg = −3.7 mm Hg (rounded to −4 mm Hg). 1 mm Hg = 1.36 cm H_2O. **(B) Breathing pressures.** Diagram of the various pressures involved in breathing. The transthoracic pressure (P_{rs}) is the pressure across the entire respiratory system. The transpulmonary pressure (P_L) is the pressure across the lung. FRC–functional residual capacity; LF–lung volume; P_A—alveolar pressure; P_{IP}—intrapleural pressure.

than P_{atm}, the P_A is said to be **positive.** When P_A is less than P_{atm}, the P_A is said to be **negative.**

3. **Intrapleural pressure (P_{IP})** is the pressure within the pleural cavity lying between the chest wall and lung. At rest, an equilibrium exists between the outward expanding force on the chest wall and an inward collapsing force on the lung. As a result of these two opposing forces, P_{IP} is **negative (−4 mm Hg or −5 cm H_2O).**

C. **Clinical consideration.** An **open pneumothorax** occurs when the parietal pleura is pierced and the pleural cavity is opened to the outside atmosphere. This causes a loss of the negative P_{IP} because P_{IP} now equals P_{atm} (P_{IP} changes from −4 mm Hg → +760 mm Hg). This results in the **expanded chest wall** (its natural tendency) and a **collapsed lung** (its natural tendency).

 Elastance

Elastance of the lung is the collapsing force that develops in the lung as the lung expands. Elastance always acts to collapse the lung. One can think of elastance as the collapsing force that builds up in a balloon completely inflated with air. The components that contribute to elastance are:

A. **Collagen and elastic fibers** within the lung (minor component)

B. **Surface tension of the alveoli** (major component)
    1. Surface tension is created at the air/surfactant interface. The relationship between elastance and surface tension is describe by the **Laplace law** below:

$$E = \frac{2T}{r}$$

where,

        E = collapsing force (elastance)

        T = surface tension

        r = radius of alveolus

The Laplace law indicates that:
    a. **Large alveoli (↑r)** have a low collapsing force (elastance) and are easy to keep open.
    b. **Small alveoli (↓r)** have a high collapsing force (elastance) and are difficult to keep open.
    2. **Surfactant** is a surface-active detergent that consists of **phosphatidylcholine** (mainly **dipalmitoyl lecithin**) and **surfactant proteins A, B, and C** produced by **type II pneumocytes.** Surfactant lines alveoli and reduces surface tension and therefore prevents collapse of small alveoli (atelectasis).

 Compliance of the Lung *(Fig. 5-3A)*

Compliance of the lung is the change in lung volume (ΔLV) divided by the change in intrapleural pressure (ΔP_{IP}) given by the equation below. Or, compliance of the lung is the slope of the line between any two points on a **pressure–volume curve.** One can think of compliance as describing the **distensibility** of the lung (or the ease at which a balloon can be inflated with air). Compliance of the lung is **increased** in obstructive lung diseases (e.g., emphysema) and compliance is **decreased** in restrictive lung diseases (e.g., idiopathic pulmonary fibrosis):

$$C = \frac{\Delta LV}{\Delta P_{IP}}$$

where,

C   = compliance

ΔLV = change in lung volume

ΔP_{IP} = change in intrapleural pressure

Ⓥ Flow–Volume Curves (Fig. 5-3B)

A flow-volume curve is generated by having an individual inspire maximally to total lung capacity (TLC) and then exhale to residual volume (RV) forcibly, rapidly, and as completely as possible.

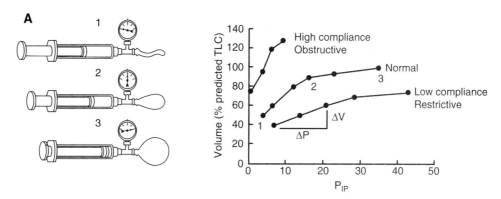

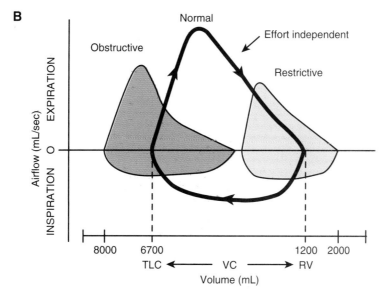

FIGURE 5-3. (A) Compliance. A simple way to visualize compliance is inflating a balloon and measuring the pressure. For each change in pressure (*1, 2, 3;* note change in syringe and manometer), the balloon inflates to a new volume, so that compliance can be defined as the slope of the line ($\Delta V/\Delta P$) between any two points on a pressure–volume curve. In a lung with normal compliance, for a given change in intrapleural pressure a certain amount of air will enter the lung. In a lung with low compliance (as seen in restrictive lung diseases), for a given change in intrapleural pressure less air will flow into the lung. In a lung with high compliance (as seen in obstructive lung diseases), for a given change in intrapleural pressure more air will flow into the lung. **(B) Flow–volume curve.** A normal maximal flow–volume curve is shown (*thick line*). Note that the air flow rises rapidly at the beginning of expiration near the total lung capacity (TLC = 6700 mL). Then, air flow decreases linearly as lung volume decreases to residual volume (RV = 1200 mL), which is called the effort independent phase. During the effort independent phase, no matter how hard the individual tries (i.e., effort), he or she will be unable to change this part of the curve. This occurs because during forced expiration, high intrathoracic pressures (5–10 times above resting) place airways under considerable pressure. If the airways are histologically normal, the airways will become somewhat compressed (but remain patent) during forced expiration and thereby limit airflow. Vital capacity (VC) equals TLC minus RV. In obstructive lung diseases, the flow–volume curve is shifted to the left as the TLC and RV are both increased. If airways are histologically abnormal as a result of a disease process (e.g., emphysema), during a forced expiration the high intrathoracic pressures will significantly compress the airways and significantly reduce the airway diameter. In severe cases, the airways may completely collapse during forced expiration and cause air trapping. In restrictive lung diseases, the flow–volume curve is shifted to the right as the TLC and RV are both decreased.

Alveolar-Blood Gas Exchange

Partial Pressure

Partial Pressure (P) *(Table 5-1)* of a gas in air is described by the **Dalton Law** as given below:

$$P = P_{atm} \times F_{gas}$$

where,

P = partial pressure

P_{atm} = atmospheric pressure (760 mm Hg)

P_{water} = partial pressure of water (47 mm Hg)

F_{gas} = fractional gas concentration; the composition of air is:
$N_2 = 78\%$, $O_2 = 21\%$, $CO_2 = \approx 0\%$

Air Flow

Air flow through the lung from the bronchi to alveoli is inversely proportional to airway resistance.

A. Airway resistance is described by the **Poiseuille law** as shown below:

$$R = \frac{8nl}{\pi r^4}$$

where,

R = resistance

n = viscosity of inspired gas

l = length of airway

r = radius of airway

Note the strong relationship of r to R. If airway radius (r) is reduced by a factor of 2, then airway resistance (R) is increased by a factor of 16 (2^4). Therefore, air flow will be dramatically reduced.

TABLE 5-1	PARTIAL PRESSURES OF O_2 AND CO_2	
Dry air	$P_{O2} = 160$ mm Hg	$P_{O2} = 760$ mm Hg $\times 0.21 = 160$
	$P_{CO2} = 0$	$P_{CO2} = 760$ mm Hg $\times 0.0 = 0$
Inspired humidified air	$P_{IO2} = 150$ mm Hg	$P_{O2} = (760 - 47$ mm Hg$) \times 0.21 = 150$
	$P_{ICO2} = 0$	$P_{CO2} = 760$ mm Hg $\times 0.0 = 0$
Alveolar air	$P_{AO2} = 100$ mm Hg	O_2 diffuses from alveoli $\rightarrow$ capillary blood
	$P_{ACO2} = 40$ mm Hg	CO_2 diffuses from capillary blood $\rightarrow$ alveoli
Systemic arterial blood	$P_{aO2} = 95$ mm Hg	Blood has equilibrated with alveolar air
	$P_{aCO2} = 40$ mm Hg	P_{O2} is <100 mm Hg because of the physiologic shunt*
Mixed venous blood	$P_{vO2} = 40$ mm Hg	O_2 has diffused from arterial blood $\rightarrow$ tissues
	$P_{vCO2} = 46$ mm Hg	CO_2 has diffused from tissues $\rightarrow$ venous blood

*See Section VA below.

B. The **medium-sized bronchi** are the **main site of airway resistance** through the contraction or relaxation of bronchial smooth muscle.

    1. **Parasympathetic stimulation, leukotrienes (LTC$_4$, LTD$_4$), PGF$_{2a}$, and thromboxane (TXA$_2$)** constrict the airways (i.e., reduce r) and thereby increase airway resistance (R). These are bronchoconstrictors.

    2. **Sympathetic stimulation, PGE$_2$, and β$_2$-adrenergic agonists (e.g., Terbutaline, Albuterol, Metaproterenol, Salmeterol)** dilate the airways (i.e., increase r) and thereby decrease airway resistance (R). These are bronchodilators.

 Blood-Air Barrier (see Histology section)

The components of the blood-air barrier are the: **surfactant layer, type I pneumocyte, basement membrane**, and **capillary endothelial cell.**

 Rate of Diffusion (RD) of O$_2$ and CO$_2$

The rate of diffusion across the blood-air barrier is governed by the **Fick law** indicated below:

$$RD = \frac{A}{T} \times D \times \left(P_1 - P_2\right)$$

where,

    A   = surface area of alveoli

    T   = thickness of blood-air barrier

    D   = solubility of the gas

    $P_1 - P_2$ = pressure difference across blood-air barrier

Note that increases in the surface area of alveoli, solubility of gas, and pressure difference will increase the rate of diffusion of O$_2$ and CO$_2$ across the blood-air barrier. However, increases in the thickness of the blood-air barrier will decrease the rate of diffusion of O$_2$ and CO$_2$ across the blood-air barrier.

 Alveolar-Arterial Gradient

The alveolar-arterial (A-a) gradient is the difference between the alveolar P$_{O2}$ (P$_{AO2}$ = A) and arterial P$_{O2}$ (P$_{aO2}$ = a). The A-a gradient indicates how well O$_2$ is equilibrating across the blood-air barrier.

A. **Normal condition.** In a normal lung, P$_{AO2}$ = 100 mm Hg and P$_{aO2}$ = 95 mm Hg (Table 5-2) such that the **A-a gradient = 100−95 = 5.** This is due to the fact that normally **2% of cardiac output** bypasses alveolar ventilation caused almost exclusively by the **bronchial circulation** (i.e., deoxygenated bronchial venous blood drains into oxygenated pulmonary venous blood; called **venous admixture**). This is referred to as a right-to-left **physiologic shunt.**

TABLE 5-2	RELATIONSHIP BETWEEN V̇$_A$, P$_{ACO2}$, AND P$_{AO2}$		
	Alveolar Ventilation Equation	**Alveolar Gas Equation**	**pH**
Hyperventilation (↑V̇$_A$)	P$_{ACO2}$ = 20 mm Hg P$_{aCO2}$ = 20 mm Hg	P$_{AO2}$ = 126 mm Hg P$_{aO2}$ = 126 mm Hg	>7.45 alkalosis
Normal V̇$_A$	P$_{ACO2}$ = 40 mm Hg* P$_{aCO2}$ = 40 mm Hg*	P$_{AO2}$ = 101 mm Hg P$_{aO2}$ = 101 mm Hg	7.3–7.4
Hypoventilation (↓V̇$_A$)	P$_{ACO2}$ = 80 mm Hg P$_{aCO2}$ = 80 mm Hg	P$_{AO2}$ = 54 mm Hg P$_{aO2}$ = 54 mm Hg	<7.35 acidosis

*See Table 5-1

B. **Tetralogy of Fallot** is a congenital heart condition such that there is skewed development of the aorticopulmonary (AP) septum. This results in a condition characterized by: **pulmonary stenosis, overriding aorta, interventricular (IV) septal defect,** and **right ventricular hypertrophy.** The resultant right-to-left shunt of blood leads to a decrease in P_{aO2} ($P_{aO2} = 40$ mm Hg) and cyanosis. The **A-a gradient = 100−40 = 60.** The dramatic increase in the A-a gradient (60 versus 5) is because approximately 50% of the cardiac output bypasses alveolar ventilation in tetralogy of Fallot.

Ⅵ Ventilation

A. **Total (or minute) ventilation ($\dot{V}_{total}$)** is the total volume of air moved in or out of the respiratory system per minute.

Normally,

$$\dot{V}_{total} = \text{tidal volume} \times \text{breaths/min}$$
$$= 500 \text{ mL} \times 15 \text{ breaths/min}$$
$$= 7500 \text{ mL/min}$$

B. **Alveolar ventilation ($\dot{V}_A$)** is the volume of air moved in or out of the alveoli per minute.

Normally,

$$\dot{V}_A = \left(\text{tidal volume} - \text{dead space}\right) \times \text{breaths/min}$$
$$= \left(500 \text{ mL} - 150 \text{ mL}\right) \times 15 \text{ breaths/min}$$
$$= 350 \text{ mL} \times 15 \text{ breaths/min}$$
$$= 5250 \text{ mL/min}$$

C. **Alveolar ventilation equation.** This equation describes the most important relationship in pulmonary physiology, which is the **inverse relationship between alveolar ventilation ($\dot{V}_A$) and P_{ACO2}** and by inference P_{aCO2}, since $P_{ACO2} = P_{aCO2}$ in a normal lung. This equation indicates that **CO_2 is the controlled variable for the regulation of ventilation.**

$$\dot{V}_A = \dot{V}_{CO2} \times K, \text{where,}$$

$\dot{V}_A$ = alveolar ventilation

$\dot{V}_{CO2}$ = rate of CO_2 production

P_{ACO2} or P_{aCO2} K = constant (0.863)

P_{ACO2} = alveolar P_{CO2}

P_{aCO2} = arterial P_{CO2}

D. **Alveolar gas equation.** This equation allows one to calculate the alveolar P_{O2} (P_{AO2}) as long as the alveolar P_{CO2} (P_{ACO2}) is known.

$$P_{AO2} = P_{IO2} - \frac{P_{ACO2}\left(F_{IO2} + 1 - F_{IO2}\right)}{R}$$

where,

P_{IO2} = P_{O2} in inspired gas

F_{IO2} = fractional concentration of O_2 in inspired gas

R   = respiratory exchange ratio (0.8)

A healthy individual who is breathing room air and has a measured $P_{aO2} = 40$ mm Hg (which closely approximates the P_{ACO2}), a barometric pressure of 760 mm Hg, and water vapor pressure of 47 mm Hg. Hence,

$$P_{AO2} = \left[(760 - 47) \times 0.21\right] - 40\left[0.21 + (1 - 0.21)/0.8\right]$$
$$= 149 - 48$$
$$= 101 \text{ mm Hg}$$

E.   Relationship between $\dot{V}_A$, P_{ACO2}, and P_{AO2} (Table 5-2). The alveolar ventilation equation and alveolar gas equation are important in assessing hyperventilation and hypoventilation states as indicated below. **Hyperventilation** is ventilation in excess of metabolic needs and may be caused by: infections, drugs, hormones (e.g., progesterone), anxiety, and exercise. **Hypoventilation** is ventilation less than metabolic needs and may be caused by: depression of the central nervous system (e.g., anesthesia, head trauma), respiratory muscle disease, thoracic cage deformities, scleroderma, and obstructive or restrictive pulmonary disease. Note that the alveolar ventilation equation demonstrates the inverse relationship between alveolar ventilation ($\dot{V}_A$) and P_{ACO2}. Note that the alveolar gas equation demonstrates the direct relationship between alveolar ventilation ($\dot{V}_A$) and P_{AO2}.

VII Pulmonary Perfusion

Pulmonary perfusion ($\dot{Q}$) is the blood flow through the lung. Pulmonary arterial blood pressure is much lower than systemic arterial blood pressure (15 mm Hg versus 100 mm Hg, respectively). **Hypoxic vasoconstriction** is a clinically important phenomenon that is unique to pulmonary circulation. If a local decrease in P_{AO2} occurs, a local vasoconstriction is produced that diverts blood flow away from the hypoxic region toward well-ventilated regions of the lung.

VIII Ventilation/Perfusion Ratio ($\dot{V}_A/\dot{Q}$) (Fig. 5-4A)

In the normal condition, the $\dot{V}_A/\dot{Q}$ ratio equals 0.8, assuming that alveolar ventilation $\dot{V}_A = 4$ L/min and pulmonary blood flow $\dot{Q} = 5$ L/min. There are two important clinical conditions that involve the $\dot{V}_A/\dot{Q}$ ratio, as indicated below:

A.   Airway blockage (e.g., child swallows a small toy). If V_A is blocked and blood flow is normal, then the **$\dot{V}_A/\dot{Q}$ ratio equals 0 (no gas exchange).** As a result, P_{aO2} and P_{aCO2} values will approach P_{vO2} and P_{vCO2} values.

B.   Blood flow blockage (e.g., pulmonary embolism). If V_A is normal and blood flow is blocked, then the **$\dot{V}_A/\dot{Q}$ ratio equals infinity (no gas exchange).** As a result, P_{AO2} and P_{ACO2} values will approach P_{IO2} and P_{ICO2} (see Table 5-1).

IX Apex Versus Base of the Lung (Fig. 5-4B)

There are regional lung differences in both $\dot{V}_A$ and $\dot{Q}$, which are both **gravity-dependent.**

A. $\dot{V}_A$ differences. In an upright individual, the lung does *not* hang from the trachea or sit on the diaphragm. Instead, each level of lung is suspended by the lung level above it. As the mass of lung that must be suspended increases, the weight of the lung pulling down or away from the chest wall will increase, thereby creating a gradient in intrapleural pressure (P_{IP}).

1.   At the lung apex, P_{IP} is decreased (more negative; **−10cm H$_2$O**). Recall that transpulmonary pressure $P_L = P_A - P_{IP}$. It follows then that the P_L at the apex will be increased. This results in **larger diameter alveoli at the apex.**

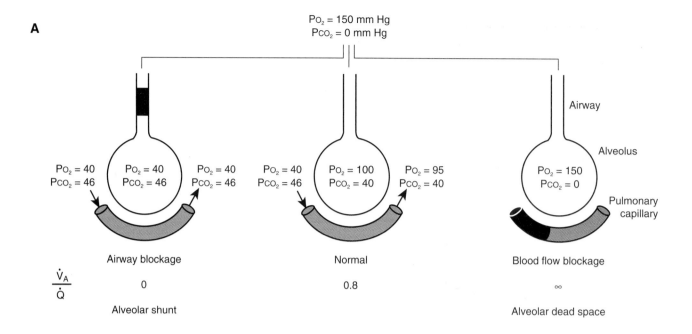

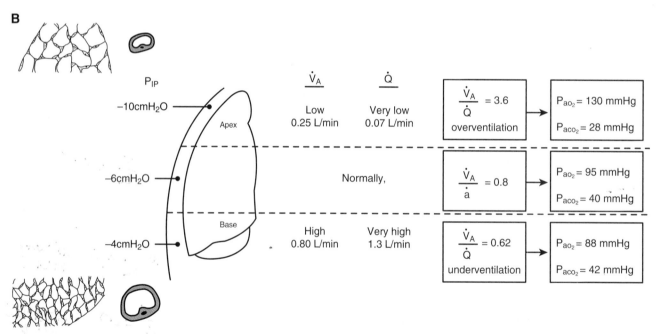

FIGURE 5-4. (A) Blockage sites. Diagram of three lung units comprised of an alveolus and capillary. All units receive the same inspired gas and mixed venous blood. The *blackened areas* indicate blockage sites in the airway and capillary. In the airway blockage, the respiratory unit receives no ventilation ($\dot{V}_A = 0$) so that the $\dot{V}_A/\dot{Q} = 0$, which is also called an alveolar shunt. An alveolar shunt occurs when a portion of the cardiac output goes through the pulmonary capillaries but does not contact alveolar air. In the blood flow blockage, the respiratory unit receives no blood flow ($\dot{Q} = 0$) so that the $\dot{V}_A/\dot{Q} = \infty$, which is also called an alveolar dead space. **(B) Apex versus base of lung.** Apex: $\dot{V}_A$ and $\dot{Q}$ are lower at the apex of the lung than at the base. Even though $\dot{V}_A$ is low, it is still too high for the very low Q. Hence, $\dot{V}_A/\dot{Q} = 3$ (overventilation or wasted ventilation) and gas exchange is more efficient. Organisms that thrive in a high O_2 environment (e.g., *Mycobacterium* tuberculosis) will flourish in the apex of the lung. During inspiration at the apex, the P_{IP} decreases from −10 to −13 cm H_2O. But because the alveoli at the apex have a large diameter (i.e., almost completely inflated before inspiration begins), very little room air flows into these alveoli. Hence, $\dot{V}_A$ is low (0.25 L/min). Base: $\dot{V}_A$ and $\dot{Q}$ are higher at the base of the lung than at the apex. Even though $\dot{V}_A$ is high, it is not high enough for the very high $\dot{Q}$. Hence, $\dot{V}_A/\dot{Q} = 0.6$ (underventilation or wasted perfusion) and gas exchange is less efficient. During inspiration at the base, the P_{IP} decreases from −2 to −5 cm H_2O. Since the alveoli at the base have a small diameter (i.e., almost completely deflated before inspiration begins), a large amount of room air flows into these alveoli. Hence, $\dot{V}_A$ is high (0.80 L/min).

2. At the lung base, P_{IP} is increased (more positive; **−4cm H_2O**). Recall that transpulmonary pressure $P_L = P_A − P_{IP}$. It follows then that the P_L at the base will be decreased. This results in **smaller diameter alveoli at the base.**

B. **Q̇ Differences.** In an upright individual, there are regional differences in blood flow through the lung caused by gravity.
   1. At the lung apex, pulmonary arterial pressure is decreased. This results in **smaller diameter blood vessels at the apex.**
   2. At the lung base, pulmonary arterial pressure is increased. This results in **larger diameter blood vessels at the base.**

X Five Causes of Hypoxemia (Fig. 5-5)

A. **Hypoventilation (↑P_{ACO2})** causes hypercapnia and hypoxemia. Hypoxemia resulting from hypoventilation can be corrected by oxygen therapy. Causes of hypoventilation include:
   1. **Primary hypoventilation** is the result of **CNS dysfunction** [e.g., narcotics, myxedema, brain damage, trauma, or central hypoventilation (Ondine curse) often seen in obese patients, sometimes called obesity hypoventilation syndrome].
   2. **Secondary hypoventilation** is the result of **PNS** or **neuromuscular dysfunction** (e.g., polio, Guillain-Barré syndrome, myasthenia gravis, Duchenne muscular dystrophy, kyphoscoliosis, or sleep apnea).
   3. **Obstructive or restrictive lung disease**

B. **V̇/Q̇ mismatch. This is a common cause of hypoxemia. V̇/Q̇ mismatch** causes hypoxemia but not necessarily hypercapnia because of a reflexive increased ventilation. Hypoxemia resulting from a V̇/Q̇ mismatch can be corrected by oxygen therapy. Causes of V/Q mismatch include:
   1. **Airway blockage (increased alveolar shunt)**
   2. **Blood flow blockage (increased alveolar dead space)**

C. **Diffusion impairment.** This is the rarest of the five causes of hypoxemia, whereby O_2 cannot diffuse from the alveoli to the capillary blood. Hypoxemia resulting from diffusion impairment can be corrected by oxygen therapy. Causes of diffusion impairment include:
   1. **Increased diffusion path** (e.g., idiopathic pulmonary fibrosis)
   2. **Decreased transit time** (e.g., ↑cardiac output, anemia)

D. **Right → left blood shunt.** Hypoxemia caused by a right-left shunt **cannot** be overcome by oxygen therapy. Causes of a right-left shunt include:
   1. **Pulmonary edema**
   2. **Pneumonia**
   3. **Heart septal defects**
   4. **Chronic liver disease**

E. **Low inspired P_{O2}.** This occurs as a result of ascent to a **high altitude.** Hypoxemia resulting from low inspired P_{O2} can be corrected by oxygen therapy.

XI Summary Diagram (Fig. 5-6)

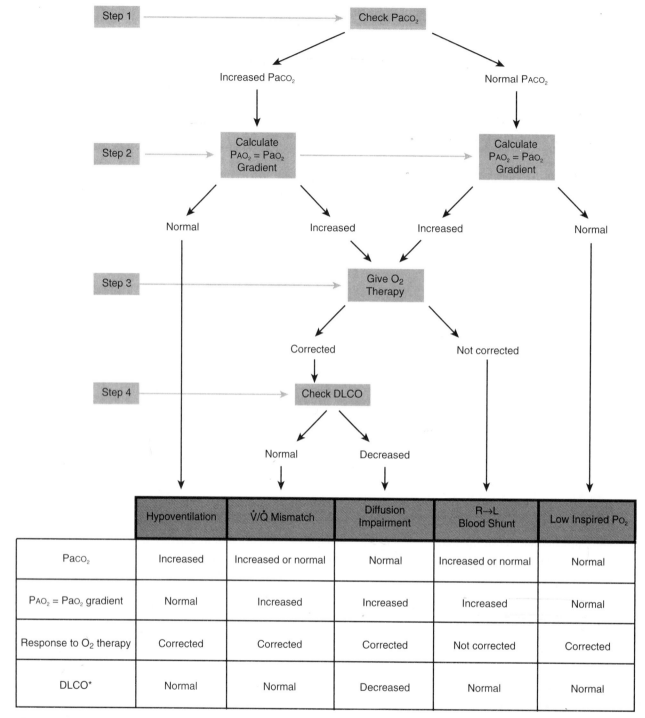

	Hypoventilation	V̇/Q̇ Mismatch	Diffusion Impairment	R→L Blood Shunt	Low Inspired P_{O_2}
Pa_{CO_2}	Increased	Increased or normal	Normal	Increased or normal	Normal
$P_{AO_2} = Pa_{O_2}$ gradient	Normal	Increased	Increased	Increased	Normal
Response to O_2 therapy	Corrected	Corrected	Corrected	Not corrected	Corrected
DLCO*	Normal	Normal	Decreased	Normal	Normal

* Diffusion-limited carbon monoxide (a measurement of diffusion capacity)

FIGURE 5-5. Differential diagnosis of hypoxemia.

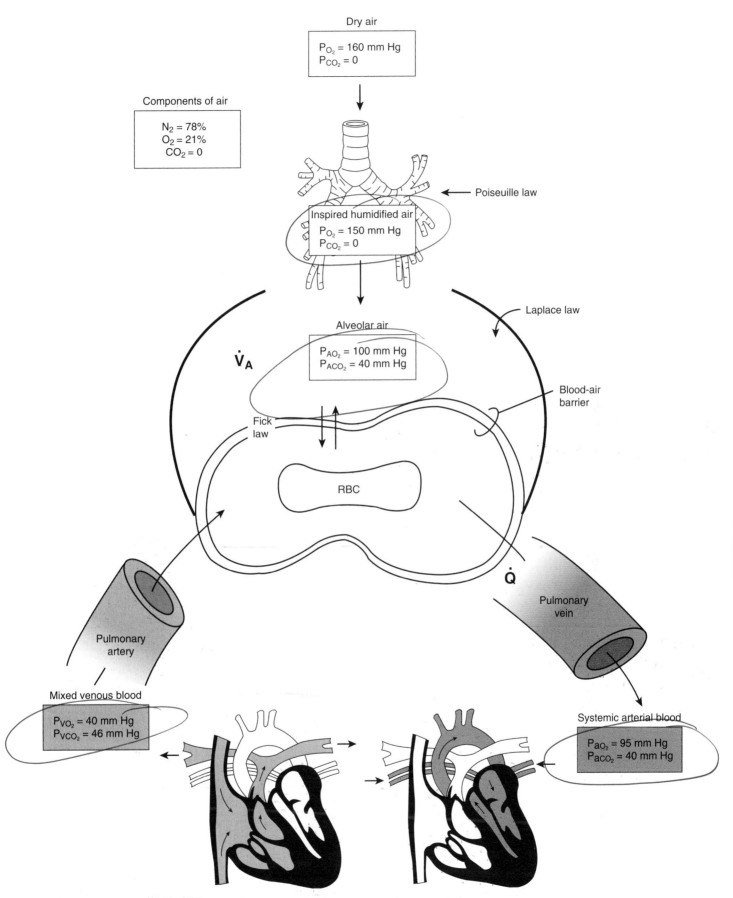

FIGURE 5-6. Airflow versus blood flow. Diagram shows the air flow ($\dot{V}_A$) through the lung and its relationship to blood flow (Q) at the blood-air barrier. Q–blood flow; RBC—red blood cells.

Transport of Oxygen and Carbon Dioxide

I Transport of Oxygen

O_2 is transported in blood in two forms:

A. **O_2 dissolved in blood.** The amount of O_2 dissolved in blood is **0.3mL O_2/dL blood** (at a P_{O_2} of 100 mm Hg; arterial blood). Hence, O_2 is not very soluble in blood.

B. **O_2 bound to hemoglobin (Hb).** The amount of O_2 bound to Hb is **19.7 mL O_2/dL blood** (at a P_{O_2} of 100 mm Hg; arterial blood).

II Total O_2 Content of Arterial Blood

$$\text{Total } O_2 \text{ content} = \text{dissolved } O_2 + O_2 \text{ bound to Hb}$$
$$= 0.3 \text{ mL } O_2/\text{dL blood} + 19.7 \text{ mL } O_2/\text{dL blood}$$
$$= \mathbf{20.0 \text{ mL } O_2/\text{dL blood}}$$

III Hemoglobin (Hb)

A. Is a globular protein consisting of four subunits.

[handwritten left margin: HbA 2α2β   HbF 2α2γ (ø2,3 BPG)]

1. **Adult Hb (HbA)** consists of two α-globin subunits and two α-globin subunits designated **Hb $\alpha_2\beta_2$.**
2. **Fetal Hb (HbF)** consists of two α-globin subunits and two γ-globin subunits designated **Hb $\alpha_2\gamma_2$.** HbF is the major form of Hb during **fetal development,** since the O_2 affinity of HbF is higher than the O_2 affinity of HbA and thereby "pulls" O_2 from the maternal blood into fetal blood. The higher O_2 affinity of HbF is explained by **2,3 bisphosphoglycerate (BPG).** When 2,3 BPG binds HbA, the O_2 affinity of HbA is lowered. However, 2,3 BPG does not bind HbF and therefore O_2 affinity of HbF is higher.

B. Contains a **heme** moiety, which is an **iron (Fe)-containing porphyrin.** Fe^{+2} (ferrous state) binds O_2 forming **oxyhemoglobin.** Fe^{+3} (ferric state) does not bind O_2 forming **deoxyhemoglobin.** The heme moiety is synthesized partially in mitochondria and partially in cytoplasm.

[handwritten left margin: Hb / 13.5–17.5 M / 12–16 F]

C. In males, the normal blood concentration of Hb is **13.5–17.5 g/dL.** In females, the normal blood concentration of Hb is **12.0–16.0 g/dL.**

D. **Clinical considerations**
1. **Thalassemia syndromes** are a heterogeneous group of genetic defects characterized by the lack of or decreased synthesis of either α-globin (**α-thalassemia**) or β-globin (**β-thalassemia**) of Hb $\alpha_2\beta_2$.
   a. **Hydrops fetalis** is the most severe form of α-thalassemia. It causes severe pallor, generalized edema, massive hepatosplenomegaly, and invariably leads to intrauterine fetal death.
   b. **β-thalassemia major** is the most severe form of β-thalassemia. It causes a severe, transfusion-dependent anemia. It is most common in Mediterranean countries and in parts of Africa and Southeast Asia.
2. **Type 1 and 2 diabetes.** The amount of **glycosylated Hb (HbA_{1c})** is an indicator of blood glucose normalization over the previous three months (since the half-life of RBCs is three months) in type 1 and type 2 diabetes. Long periods of elevated

[handwritten bottom: 120 days = 3 mos]

blood glucose levels will result in a glycosylated Hb of 12–20%, whereas normal levels are approximately 5%.

Ⅳ   Hemoglobin-O₂ Dissociation Curve *(Fig. 5-7A)*

Each Hb molecule can carry up to **four O₂** molecules. A Hb-O₂ dissociation curve is **sigmoid-shaped** because each successive O₂ that binds to Hb increases the affinity for the next O₂ (called **positive cooperativity**). Hence, the affinity for the fourth O₂ is the highest. There are three important points on the curve, as follows:

A.   **PO₂ = 25 mm Hg.** At this point, Hb is **50% saturated** (called the **P₅₀**). This means that Hb is bound to two O₂ molecules.

B.   **PO₂ = 75 mm Hg (venous blood).** At this point, Hb is **75% saturated.** This means that Hb is bound to three O₂ molecules.

C.   **PO₂ = 100 mm Hg (arterial blood).** At this point, Hb is almost **100% saturated.** This means that Hb is bound to four O₂ molecules.

(handwritten margin note:) $P_{50} = 25\,mmHg$

Ⅴ   Shifts in the Hemoglobin-O₂ Dissociation Curve *(Fig. 5-7, B and C)*

A.   **A shift to the left** occurs when the **affinity of Hb for O₂** is increased. This makes the unloading of O₂ from arterial blood to tissues more difficult. A shift to the left is caused by a number of different factors:
   1.   **Decreased P_{aCO2}, increased arterial pH** (e.g., alkalosis)
   2.   **Decreased body temperature**
   3.   **Decreased 2,3-BPG** (e.g., stored blood, HbF). Stored blood loses 2,3-BPG. HbF does not bind 2,3-BPG.

B.   **A shift to the right** occurs when the **affinity of Hb for O₂ is decreased.** This makes the unloading of O₂ from arterial blood to tissues easier. A shift to the right is caused by a number of different factors:
   1.   **Increased P_{aCO2}, decreased arterial pH** (e.g., acidosis)
   2.   **Increased body temperature** (e.g., exercise)
   3.   **Increased 2,3 BPG** (e.g., living at high altitude)

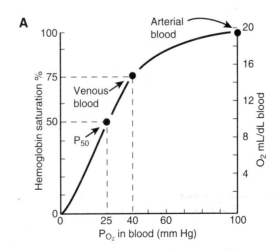

FIGURE 5-7. (A) Hemoglobin-O₂ dissociation curve. P_{O2} in the blood usually is measured by an oxygen electrode in blood taken by a puncture of the radial artery (i.e., arterial P_{O2}). Generally, arterial P_{CO2} and arterial pH are measured at the same time. Normal ranges are: arterial P_{O2} = 75–105 mm Hg, arterial P_{CO2} = 33–45 mm Hg, arterial pH = 7.35–7.45, serum HCO₃⁻ = 22–28 mEq/L. Whenever you read a report of arterial P_{O2}, you should recall the hemoglobin-O₂ dissociation curve. Remember the three anchor points on the curve: P_{O2} = 25 mm Hg (the P₅₀), P_{O2} = 40 mm Hg (venous blood), and P_{O2} = 100 mm Hg (arterial blood) as indicated. Also note that the curve is flat between P_{O2} = 60–100 mm Hg, which means that humans can tolerate relatively large changes in P_{O2} without changing the oxygen-carrying capacity of Hb.

(continued)

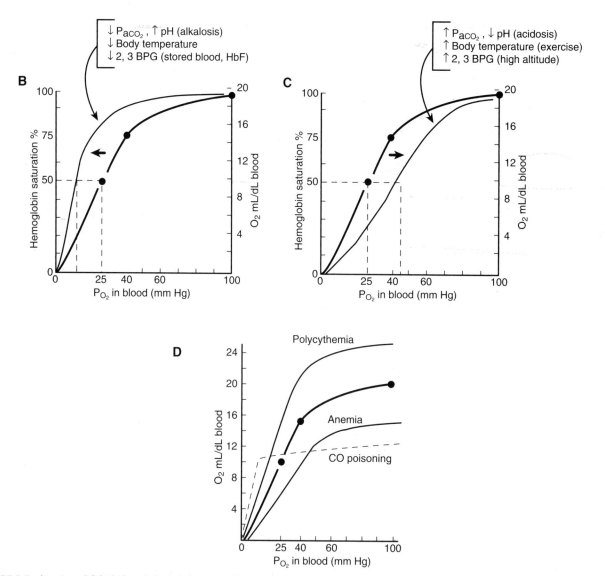

FIGURE 5-7. *(continued)* **(B) Shift to left.** A shift to the left of the hemoglobin-O_2 dissociation curve. Note the various factors that cause a shift to the left and that the P_{50} is decreased. **(C) Shift to right.** A shift to the right of the hemoglobin-O_2 dissociation curve. Note the various factors that cause a shift to the right and that the P_{50} is increased. **(D) Polycythemia, anemia, and carbon monoxide (CO) poisoning.** In polycythemia, the O_2 content of the blood is above normal (24 versus 20 mL of O_2/dL blood) because of the increased Hb concentration. In anemia, the O_2 content of the blood is below normal (14 versus 20 mL of O_2/dL blood) because of the decreased Hb concentration. In CO poisoning, the O_2 content of the blood is below normal (12 versus 20 mL of O_2/dL blood) because CO binds to Hb with a high affinity taking up O_2 sites. In addition, CO poisoning causes a shift to the left of the curve. Note that the main change in these curves compared with normal is at the plateau or the total O_2-carrying capacity of the blood. BPG—bisphosphoglycerate.

Ⓥ️ⓘ Clinical Considerations *(Fig. 5-7D)*

A. Polycythemia vera is myeloproliferative disorder whereby the RBC precursors dominate and result in an increased RBC mass.

B. Anemia

1. **Iron-deficiency anemia** (most common type of anemia) reduces **heme synthesis.** This deficiency is the result of inadequate iron intake or absorption (e.g., dietary deficiency, celiac disease), excessive iron loss (e.g., menstruation, gastrointestinal bleeding), or increased iron demand (e.g., pregnancy, infancy). Clinical findings include: RBCs are microcytic, hypochromatic, and cigar-shaped with a thin rim of Hb at the periphery; low serum ferritin levels (<12 ug/L; normal range: 15–200

ug/L) and low serum iron levels (250 ug/L; normal range: 500–1700 ug/L); high total iron binding capacity (6000 ug/L; normal value: 3000 ug/L); and low transferrin saturation (10%; normal value: 30%).

2. **Vitamin B_{12} (pernicious anemia) and folate deficiency** reduce **DNA synthesis** in hematopoietic stem cells, thereby hindering erythropoiesis. These nutritional deficiencies are a result of malabsorption of vitamin B_{12} (e.g., type A gastritis, which destroys **parietal cells** of the stomach that secrete **intrinsic factor** necessary for absorption of vitamin B_{12} from the ileum); low intake of folic acid (e.g., alcoholism); increased demand for folic acid (e.g., pregnancy; folic acid is also necessary to prevent neural tube defects in the fetus); and methotrexate chemotherapy. Clinical findings include: RBCs are macrocytic, hyperchromatic, and teardrop-shaped (dacryocysts); neutrophils with a hypersegmented nucleus; bone marrow contains numerous megaloblasts; neuropathy involving posterior white columns and corticospinal tract; low serum vitamin B_{12} levels (<100 pg/mL; normal range: 200–900 pg/mL); and low serum folate levels (<4 ng/mL; normal range 6–20 ng/mL).

C. **Carbon monoxide (CO) poisoning.** CO binds to Hb with an affinity 200-fold greater than that of O_2, forming **carboxyhemoglobin (HbCO)** that gives blood a characteristic **cherry-red color**. CO poisoning **decreases the O_2 content** of the blood and causes a **shift to the left** of the hemoglobin-O_2 dissociation curve. Patients with CO poisoning are given 100% O_2 to breath in order to competitively displace CO from Hb and to increase the amount of dissolved O_2 content in the blood.

VII Transport of Carbon Dioxide (CO_2) (Fig. 5-8). CO_2 is transported in blood in three forms:

A. **CO_2 dissolved in blood.** 5% of the total CO_2 is transported in this form.

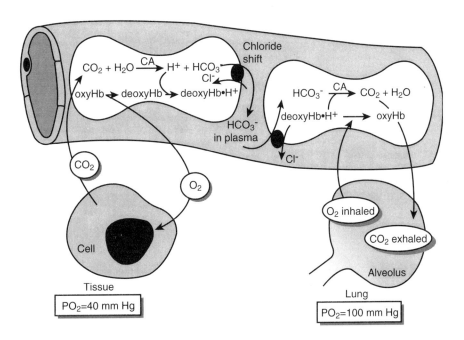

FIGURE 5-8. Blood gas exchange in tissues and lung alveoli. In tissues, CO_2 is generated and freely diffuses into RBCs. In RBCs, CO_2 combines with H_2O to form H+ and HCO_3^- that is catalyzed by **carbonic anhydrase** (CA). HCO_3^- leaves the RBC in exchange for Cl- (called the **chloride shift**) using **band III protein** (*solid black dot*). CO_2 is transported to the lung as HCO_3^- in the plasma. The P_{O2} within tissues is 40 mm Hg and favors O_2 dissociation from oxyHb to form deoxyHb. The O_2 freely diffuses to tissues. The H+ is buffered by combining with deoxyHb to form deoxyHb.H+. In the lung, HCO_3^- enters the RBC and combines with H+ from deoxyHb.H+ to form CO_2 and H_2O. This reaction is catalyzed by carbonic anhydrase (CA). CO_2 diffuses to lung alveoli and is exhaled. The P_{O2} within lung alveoli is 100 mm Hg and favors saturation of deoxyHb with O_2 to form oxyHb.

B. CO$_2$ bound to Hb (HbCO$_2$; carbaminohemoglobin). 5% of the total CO$_2$ is transported in this form.

C. HCO$_3^-$. 90% of the total CO$_2$ is transported in this form.

Ⅷ Control of Breathing (Fig. 5-9)

The rate and depth of breathing are regulated so that arterial P$_{CO_2}$ = 40 mm Hg. Under normal circumstances, the P$_{aCO_2}$ is the major determinant of breathing and is held to within +/− 3 mm Hg. A 1–2 mm Hg increase in P$_{aCO_2}$ evokes a 30 to 40% increase in ventilation.

A. Receptors

1. **Medulla receptors** are primarily stimulated by an **increased P$_{aCO_2}$**. CO$_2$ freely crosses the blood–brain barrier to enter the cerebrospinal fluid (CSF). In the CSF,

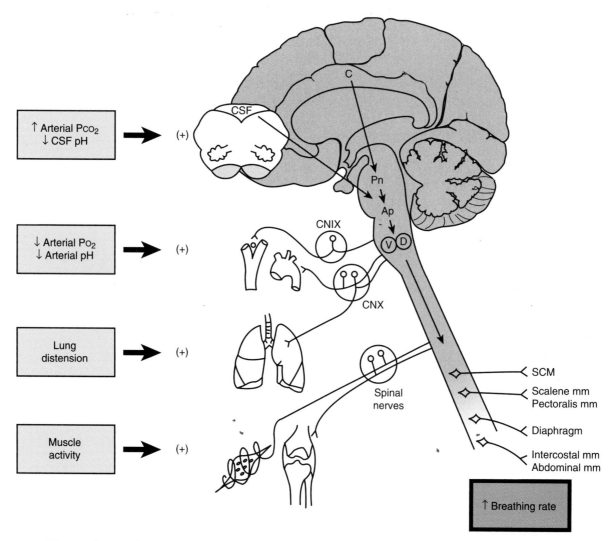

FIGURE 5-9. Diagram showing the control of breathing. The SCM muscle is innervated by cranial nerve XI (CN XI). The scalene and pectoralis muscles are innervated by cervical spinal nerves (C5–C8). The diaphragm is innervated by the phrenic nerve. The intercostals and abdominal muscles are innervated by intercostal nerves. Cell bodies of afferent nerve fibers are located in the petrosal ganglion (CN IX), nodose ganglion (CN X), and dorsal root ganglion (spinal nerves). C—cerebral cortex; CSF–cerebrospinal fluid; D—dorsal respiratory group; Pn—pneumotaxic center; Ap—apneustic center; V—ventral respiratory group; D—dorsal respiratory group in medulla; V—ventral respiratory group in medulla; SCM—sternocleidomastoid muscle.

CO_2 combines with H_2O to form H_2CO_3 (carbonic acid), which dissociates to H+ and HCO_3−. The medulla receptors sense high levels of [H+] in CSF and therefore respond to a **decrease in CSF pH (normal CSF pH = 7.32).** Note that the medulla receptors do NOT respond to O_2 at all.

2. **Carotid body and aortic bodies** are peripheral **chemoreceptors** that are primarily stimulated by a **decreased P_{aO2}** (<60 mm Hg) and a decreased **arterial pH (acidosis).** The carotid body and aortic bodies are the **only sites that detect changes in P_{aO2}.** Afferent nerve fibers of **CN IX,** whose cell bodies are located in the **petrosal ganglion,** innervate the **carotid body** and relay information to the CNS respiratory centers via the **solitary nucleus.** Afferent nerve fibers of **CN X,** whose cell bodies are located in the nodose ganglion, innervate the **aortic bodies** and relay information to the CNS respiratory centers via the **solitary nucleus.** In **diabetic ketoacidosis,** there is a decreased arterial pH (acidosis), which leads to an increased tidal volume (TV) and minute ventilation (amount of air inspired or expired each minute). This is called **Kussmaul breathing.**

3. **Stretch receptors** in the lung are stimulated by lung distension. Afferent nerve fibers of CN X via the solitary nucleus relay information to CNS respiratory centers. The **Hering–Breuer reflex** produces an apnea (absence of breathing) after large lung inflations. This reflex is very prominent in newborn infants.

4. **Muscle spindle and joint receptors** are stimulated by muscle activity. Afferent nerve fibers from these receptors relay information to CNS respiratory centers via the dorsal column-medial lemniscal pathway.

5. **Note:** In chronically hypercapnic patients, both medulla and peripheral receptors become refractory to ↑CO_2 so that the only drive to maintain respiration is hypoxemia that is sensed by the peripheral receptors. Consequently, when administering O_2 therapy to correct the hypoxemia in chronically hypercapnic patients, care must be taken because correcting the hypoxemia may lead to respiratory failure.

B. **CNS respiratory centers.** Breathing is normally a smooth, cyclic process. However, in some CNS diseases and congestive heart failure **Cheyne–Stokes breathing** is observed. Cheyne–Stokes breathing is rapid breathing of increasing (↑TV) and decreasing (↓TV) depth followed by apnea lasting 10 to 20 seconds. **Apneustic breathing** is characterized by prolonged inspirations followed by brief periods of expiration.

1. **Cerebral cortex.** A person can voluntarily control breathing.
2. **Pneumotaxic center** is located in the upper pons and inhibits inspiration.
3. **Apneustic center** is located in the lower pons and stimulates inspiration.
4. **Medulla.** The **dorsal respiratory group (DRG)** is responsible for inspiration and controls the basic rhythm for breathing. Sensory input comes from the carotid body, aortic bodies, and lung stretch receptors via afferent nerve fibers traveling with CN IX and CN X. The **ventral respiratory group (VRG)** is responsible for expiration. The VRG does not play a role during normal breathing because expiration is a passive process. However, the VRG does play a role during exercise when expiration is an active process. The **pre-Botzinger complex** is a region in the ventrolateral medulla that contains a group of pacemaker neurons responsible for respiratory rhythmogenesis. Output from the DRG and VRG modulate lower motor neurons of **cranial nerve XI, cervical spinal nerves (C5–C8), phrenic nerve, and intercostal nerves** that innervate the **sternocleidomastoid, scalene/pectoralis muscles, diaphragm, and intercostal/abdominal muscles,** respectively.

IX Physiology of High Altitude

When a person ascends from sea level (P_{atm} = 760 mm Hg) to a high altitude (P_{atm} = 400 mm Hg), the P_{O2} of humidified air decreases from 150 mm Hg to 80 mm Hg, respectively. This decreases P_{AO2} and as a result **decreases P_{aO2} (<60 mm Hg),** that is, **hypoxemia.** Hypoxemia stimulates the process as indicated in *Figure 5-10.*

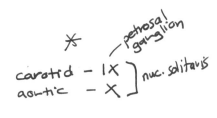

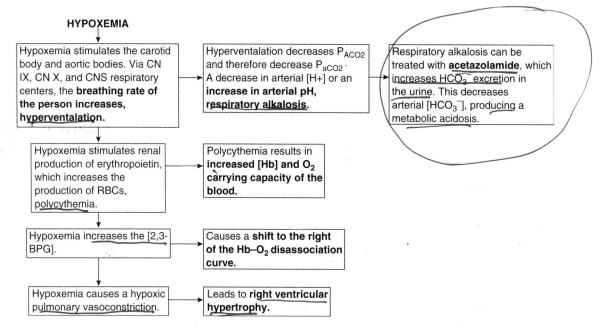

HYPOXEMIA

Hypoxemia stimulates the carotid body and aortic bodies. Via CN IX, CN X, and CNS respiratory centers, the **breathing rate of the person increases, hyperventalation.**

Hyperventalation decreases P_{ACO2} and therefore decrease P_{aCO2}. A decrease in arterial [H+] or an **increase in arterial pH, respiratory alkalosis.**

Respiratory alkalosis can be treated with **acetazolamide**, which increases HCO_3^- excretion in the urine. This decreases arterial $[HCO_3^-]$, producing a metabolic acidosis.

Hypoxemia stimulates renal production of erythropoietin, which increases the production of RBCs, polycythemia.

Polycythemia results in **increased [Hb] and O_2 carrying capacity of the blood.**

Hypoxemia increases the [2,3-BPG].

Causes a **shift to the right of the Hb–O_2 disassociation curve.**

Hypoxemia causes a hypoxic pulmonary vasoconstriction.

Leads to **right ventricular hypertrophy.**

FIGURE 5-10. Processes stimulated by hypoxemia.

Acetazolamide: ↑ bicarb excret. in urine ⟶ metab acidosis

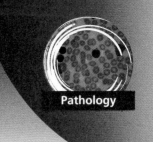

Chapter **6**

Pathology

I Atelectasis

Atelectasis is the incomplete expansion of alveoli (in neonates) or collapse of alveoli (in adults). There are four types of atelectasis, as indicated below.

A. Compression atelectasis is the mechanical collapse of alveoli caused by external pressure as a result of a pneumothorax, tumor, or pleural effusions.

B. Resorption atelectasis is the collapse of alveoli distal to an obstruction (e.g., foreign body, mucous plugs, or tumors) within a bronchus.

C. Contraction atelectasis is the focal loss of alveoli as a result of interstitial fibrosis, which prevents complete expansion of alveoli and increases elastic recoil of alveoli.

D. Microatelectasis is the generalized inability of the lung to expand as a result of the loss of surfactant, usually seen in the following conditions:
  1. **Neonatal respiratory distress syndrome (NRDS) is** caused by a deficiency of surfactant, which may occur as a result of prolonged intrauterine asphyxia, in premature infants, or in infants of diabetic mothers. Lung maturation is assessed by the **lecithin:sphingomyelin ratio** in amniotic fluid (a ratio > 2:1 = maturity). **Thyroxine** and **cortisol** treatment can increase surfactant production. Pathological findings include hemorrhagic edema within the lung, atelectasis, and **hyaline membrane disease** characterized by eosinophilic material consisting of proteinaceous fluid (fibrin, plasma) and necrotic cells. A deficiency of surfactant causes the surface tension (or attraction) to increase and therefore the elastance (or collapsing force) of the lung is increased as described by the Laplace law. The elastance is increased so much that the newborn cannot inflate the lungs with air. The newborn works harder and harder with each successive breath to try to inflate the lungs, but to no avail. The newborn develops hypoxemia, which causes pulmonary vasoconstriction, pulmonary hypoperfusion, and capillary endothelium damage.
  2. **Adult respiratory distress syndrome (ARDS)** is defined as a secondary surfactant deficiency resulting from other primary pathologies that damage either alveolar cells or capillary endothelial cells in the lung. ARDS is a clinical term for diffuse alveolar damage leading to respiratory failure. ARDS may be caused by the following: inhalation of toxic gases (e.g., 9/11 rescue workers), near-drowning water, or extremely hot air; left ventricular failure resulting in cardiogenic pulmonary edema; illicit drugs (e.g., heroin); metabolic disorders (e.g., uremia, acidosis, acute pancreatitis); severe trauma (e.g., car accident with multiple fractures); shock (e.g., endotoxins or ischemia can damage cells). A common pathological course of ARDS is as follows:
     a. As the blood-air barrier is damaged, an **active exudative process** occurs whereby fluid (edema), neutrophils, macrophages, cell debris, fibrin (inhibits synthesis of surfactant), and hyaline membranes are observed in the alveolar lumen.
     b. A **proliferative process** occurs whereby type II pneumocytes not only proliferate and differentiate into type I pneumocytes but also re-establish the synthesis of surfactant. The prognosis for return to normal lung function is good.

c. A **chronic fibrosis process** may occur if the initial damage is severe whereby fibroblasts proliferate and cause intra-alveolar fibrosis that seriously affects gas exchange.

Pulmonary Embolism

Pulmonary embolism (PE) is the occlusion of the pulmonary arteries or its branches by an embolic blood clot originating from a deep vein thrombosis (DVT) in the leg or pelvic area. A **large embolus** may occlude the main pulmonary artery or lodge at the bifurcation as a "**saddle embolus,**" which may cause sudden death with symptoms easily confused with myocardial infarction (i.e., chest pain, severe dyspnea, shock, increased serum lactate dehydrogenase [LDH] levels). A **medium-sized embolism** may occlude segmental arteries and may produce a **pulmonary infarction,** which is wedge-shaped and usually occurs in the lower lobes. A group of **small emboli ("emboli showers")** may occlude smaller peripheral branches of the pulmonary artery and cause pulmonary hypertension over time. Risk factors include: obesity, cancer, pregnancy, oral contraceptives, hypercoagulability, multiple bone fractures, burns, and prior DVT. A typical clinical scenario involves a postsurgical, bedridden patient who develops sudden shortness of breath.

Bronchiectasis

Bronchiectasis is the abnormal, permanent dilatation of bronchi as a result of chronic necrotizing infection (e.g., *Staphylococcus, Streptococcus, Haemophilus influenzae*), bronchial obstruction (e.g., foreign body, mucous plugs, or tumors), or congenital conditions (e.g., Kartagener syndrome, cystic fibrosis, immunodeficiency disorders). The **lower lobes** of the lung are predominately affected and the affected bronchi have a **saccular** appearance. Clinical signs include: cough, fever, and expectoration of large amounts of foul-smelling purulent sputum.

Obstructive Lung Diseases

Obstructive lung diseases are characterized by an **increase in airway resistance (particularly expiratory airflow). Obstructive ventilatory impairment** is the impairment of airflow during expiration with concomitant air trapping and hyperinflation. The increase in airway resistance (as a result of narrowing of the airway lumen) can be caused by conditions: **in the wall of the airway** wherein smooth muscle hypertrophy may cause airway narrowing (e.g., asthma), **outside the airway** wherein destruction of lung parenchyma may cause airway narrowing upon expiration as a result of a loss of radial traction (e.g., emphysema), and **in the lumen of the airway** wherein increased mucus production may cause airway narrowing (e.g., chronic bronchitis).

A. **Asthma**
   1. **General features.** Asthma is associated with **smooth muscle hyperactivity within bronchi and bronchioles, increased mucus production, and edema of the bronchial wall.** Patients with asthma have the following characteristics: a decreased P_{aO2} (hypoxemia) leads to stimulation of the carotid and aortic bodies and hyperventilation, a decreased P_{aCO2} (hypocapnia), and respiratory alkalosis. As the asthma attack worsens, hypoventilation occurs and leads to a further decreased P_{aO2}, a severely increased P_{aCO2} (hypercapnia), respiratory acidosis, and death.
   2. **Pathology.** Pathological findings include: inflammatory cell infiltrates containing numerous **eosinophils** within the bronchial wall, hyperplasia of bronchial smooth muscle, hypertrophy of seromucous glands, **Curschmann spirals** (formed from shed epithelium), and **Charcot-Leyden crystals** (formed from eosinophil granules) within the mucous plugs.

B. **Emphysema** is a type of **chronic obstructive pulmonary disease (COPD).** In the early stages of emphysema, there is enlargement of air spaces distal to the terminal bronchiole called **air trapping.** In the later stages of emphysema, further lung tissue and alveolar damage result in additional air trapping, which is now called **hyperinflation.** Emphysematous patients have much less difficulty inhaling air into the lung ($\uparrow$compliance) than a normal individual. However, emphysematous patients have much more difficulty exhaling air out of the lung, which increases the work of breathing (i.e., respiratory muscles), manifested by shortness of breath (dyspnea). Emphysematous patient breathe slower with large tidal volumes.

1. **General features.** Patients are referred to as "**pink puffers**" with the following characteristics: a thin, barrel-shaped chest, increased breathing rate (tachypnea), a mildly decreased P_{aO2} (mild hypoxemia), a mildly decreased or normal P_{aCO2} (hypocapnia or normocapnia), and decreased diffusion-limited carbon monoxide (DLCO).

2. **Pathology**
   a. **Centriacinar emphysema** (related to **smoking**). Pathological findings include: a widening of the air spaces within the **respiratory bronchioles** only while the surrounding alveoli remain fairly well preserved.
   b. **Panacinar emphysema** (related to α_1-**antitrypsin deficiency**). Pathological findings include: a widening of the air spaces within the **alveolar ducts, alveolar sacs,** and **alveoli** as a result of destruction of the alveolar walls by enzymes.

C. **Chronic bronchitis** is a **type of COPD** that is related to smoking.

1. **General features.** Patients are referred to as "**blue bloaters**" with the following characteristics: a muscular, barrel-shaped chest, severely decreased P_{aO2} (severe hypoxemia with cyanosis), increased P_{aCO2} (hypercapnia) leads to chronic respiratory acidosis, increased $H_2CO_3^-$ reabsorption by the kidney to buffer the acidemia, right ventricular failure, and systemic edema.

2. **Pathology.** Pathological findings include: inflammatory cell infiltrates within the bronchial wall; hypertrophy of seromucous glands (increase in Reid index); an excessive mucus production leading to copious, purulent sputum production; and recurrent inflammation, infection, and scarring in terminal airways resulting in a decrease in average small airway diameter.

V Restrictive Lung Diseases

Restrictive lung diseases are characterized by a **decrease in compliance** (i.e., the distensibility of the lung is restricted). The lungs are said to be "**stiff.**" **Restrictive ventilatory impairment** is the inability to fully expand the lung **(inspiratory airflow),** which results in a decrease in total lung capacity (TLC).

A. **Idiopathic pulmonary fibrosis**

1. **General features.** Patients with idiopathic pulmonary fibrosis have the following characteristics: a decreased P_{aO2} (hypoxemia) and a mildly decreased or normal P_{aCO2} (hypocapnia or normocapnia). **During exercise, the hypoxemia worsens without hypercapnia.** As the condition worsens, hypoventilation leads to a further decreased P_{aO2}, a severely increased P_{aCO2} (hypercapnia), respiratory acidosis, and decreased diffusion limited carbon monoxide (DLCO).

2. **Pathology.** Pathological findings include: inflammatory cell infiltrates, thickening of the blood-air barrier (i.e., alveolar wall) as a result of collagen production by fibroblasts, and destruction of alveolar architecture leading to formation of air-filled cystic spaces surrounded by thickened scar tissue (i.e., "honeycomb lung").

B. **Coal worker pneumoconiosis (CWP; "black lung disease")** results from the inhalation of **coal dust** and generally is benign with little if any reduction in lung function. The appearance of large nodular lesions suggests a change caused by silica in the inhaled dust such that the disease is now called **anthracosilicosis. Anthracosis** is the most innocuous lesion observed whereby carbon pigment is phagocytosed by alveolar macrophages that accumulate along the lymphatics. **Simple CWP** occurs when carbon pigment is phagocytosed by alveolar macrophages that organize into **coal nodules** usually found adjacent to respiratory bronchioles. **Complicated CWP** or **progressive massive fibrosis (PMF)** occurs when there is a confluent, fibrosing reaction in the lung. PMF occurs on a background of simple CWP and consists of multiple, large scars consisting of dense collagen and carbon pigment. **Caplan syndrome** is the coexistence of rheumatoid arthritis and CWP whereby distinctive pulmonary nodular lesions (similar to rheumatoid nodules) develop rapidly.

C. **Silicosis** results from the inhalation of **silicon dioxide** (silica; SiO_2) and is associated with an increased disposition to **tuberculosis** (i.e., silicotuberculosis). Silicosis is characterized by small, dense, collagenous nodules that contain birefringent silica crystals.

D. **Asbestosis** results from the inhalation of asbestos fibers. There are two geometric forms of asbestos; a **serpentine form** (curly, flexible fibers) and an **amphibole form** (straight, stiff fibers). The amphibole form is more pathogenic. Asbestosis is characterized by **diffuse pulmonary interstitial fibrosis** and **asbestos bodies.** Asbestos bodies are golden-brown, beaded rods that consist of asbestos fibers coated with iron-containing protein material. These bodies arise when alveolar macrophages attempt to phagocytose asbestos fibers. **Malignant mesothelioma** is the most serious pleural neoplasm and is associated with a history of asbestos exposure.

E. **Sarcoidosis** is a **type IV hypersensitivity** reaction to an unknown antigen. Sarcoidosis is characterized by a **noncaseating granuloma** distributed along the lymphatics in the lung. The noncaseating granuloma is an aggregation of epithelioid cells with Langerhans cells and foreign body-type giant cells, **asteroid bodies,** which are stellate inclusions bodies found within giant cells, and **Schaumann bodies,** which are laminated concretions of calcium and proteins. Sarcoidosis is common in the Southeast United States and in young black women.

F. **Hypersensitivity pneumonitis** is a general term used to describe lung disorders caused by inhalation of a variety of organic dusts. These lung disorders are a **type IV hypersensitivity** reaction that results in the formation of granulomas and fibrosis. Numerous specific syndromes have been named: **byssinosis** (a reaction to cotton or hemp fibers), **farmer's lung** (a reaction to molds in hay dust), **silo-filler's lung** (a reaction to nitrous oxides found in corn silos), **bagassosis** (a reaction to moldy sugar cane), **humidifier lung** (a reaction to thermophilic bacteria in heated water reservoirs), and **pigeon breeder's lung** (a reaction to serum, excreta, and feathers of birds).

G. **Pulmonary eosinophilia.** A number of diverse pathological pulmonary diseases are characterized by an infiltration of eosinophils due in part to interleukin-5 (IL-5). **Simple pulmonary eosinophilia (Löffler syndrome)** is characterized by thickened interalveolar septae as a result of infiltration of eosinophils and giant cells. **Tropical eosinophilia** is caused by infection with microfilariae. **Secondary chronic pulmonary eosinophilia** occurs in a number of parasitic, fungal, and bacterial infections; in hypersensitivity pneumonitis; in drug allergies; and in association with asthma and aspergillosis. **Chronic eosinophilic pneumonia** is characterized by focal areas of cellular consolidation chiefly in the lung periphery composed of lymphocytes and eosinophils within the interalveolar septae and alveoli.

H. **Bronchiolitis obliterans-organizing pneumonia (BOOP)** refers to the common response of the lungs to infection or inflammatory injury. This is characterized by plugs of loose, fibrous tissue filling bronchioles and alveoli. Chronic inflammatory cell infiltrates accompany what appears to be a prolonged effort to resolve the pulmonary injury.

I. **Diffuse pulmonary hemorrhage syndromes.** Some interstitial pulmonary disorders are accompanied by hemorrhage from the lung. These include: Goodpasture syndrome, idiopathic pulmonary hemosiderosis, and vasculitis-associated hemorrhage. **Goodpasture syndrome** is the simultaneous appearance of progressive glomerulonephritis and hemorrhagic interstitial pneumonitis as a result of the presence of antibodies evoked by antigens in both glomerular and alveolar basement membranes.

Ⅵ Obstructive Versus Restrictive *(Fig. 6-1)*

Obstructive lung diseases (e.g., asthma, emphysema, chronic bronchitis) and restrictive lung diseases (e.g., idiopathic pulmonary fibrosis) demonstrate distinct differences in various lung parameters.

Ⅶ Bronchogenic Carcinoma

Bronchogenic carcinoma begins as hyperplasia of the bronchial epithelium with continued progression occurring through intraluminal growth, infiltrative peribronchial growth, and intraparenchymal growth. Intrathoracic spread of bronchogenic carcinoma may lead to: **Horner syndrome** (miosis, ptosis, hemianhydrosis, and apparent enophthalmos) as a result of cervical sympathetic chain involvement; **SVC syndrome** causing dilatation of head and neck veins, facial swelling, and cyanosis; **dysphagia** as a result of esophageal obstruction; **hoarseness of voice** as a result of recurrent laryngeal nerve involvement; **paralysis of diaphragm** as a result of phrenic nerve involvement; and **Pancoast syndrome** causing ulnar nerve pain and Horner syndrome. Tracheobronchial, parasternal, and supraclavicular lymph nodes are involved in the lymphatic metastasis of bronchogenic carcinoma. Enlargement of the tracheobronchial nodes may **indent the esophagus,** which can be observed radiologically during a barium swallow or by **distorted position of the carina.** Metastasis to the brain via arterial blood may occur by the following route: cancer cells enter a lung capillary → pulmonary vein → left atrium and ventricle → aorta → internal carotid and vertebral arteries. Metastasis to the brain via venous blood may occur by the following route: cancer cells enter a bronchial vein → azygous vein → external and internal vertebral venous plexuses → cranial dural sinuses. As approximately 25% of primary lung cancers do not have an obvious bronchial origin, the term "bronchogenic" may not be entirely appropriate. The most important issue in primary lung cancer is the histological subclassifications, which include:

A. **Adenocarcinoma (AD)** has a 35% incidence and is the most common lung cancer in nonsmokers. AD is peripherally located within the lung, as it arises from distal airways and alveoli and forms a well-circumscribed gray–white mass. There are four major histological subtypes of AD, although it is common to find mixtures of subtypes:
    1. The **acinar subtype** (most common subtype) features cuboidal- or polygonal-shaped cells containing mucus arranged in an acinus (i.e., glandular formation).
    2. The **solid with mucus formation subtype** features cuboidal- or polygonal-shaped cells containing mucus arranged in solid cell nests. This subtype is a poorly differentiated tumor (i.e., no glandular formation as seen in the acinar subtype).
    3. The **papillary subtype** features a single layer of tall, columnar-shaped cells arranged in a papillary fashion on a core of fibrovascular connective tissue.
    4. The **bronchioloalveolar subtype** grows along pre-existing alveolar walls and is either **nonmucinous** (70%) or **mucinous** (30%). The nonmucinous pattern consists of Clara cells or type II pneumocytes. The mucinous pattern consists of tall, columnar-shaped cells containing mucus.

B. **Squamous cell carcinoma (SQ)** has a 35% incidence and is most closely associated with **smoking history.** SQ is centrally located as it arises from larger bronchi as a result of injury of the bronchial epithelium followed by regeneration from the basal layer in the form of squamous metaplasia. SQ begins as a small, red, granular plaque and progresses to a large intrabronchial mass. Cavitation of the lung may occur distal to the mass. SQ may secrete **parathyroid hormone (PTH)** causing hypercalcemia.

Normal Lung	Obstructive Lung Diseases	Restrictive Lung Diseases
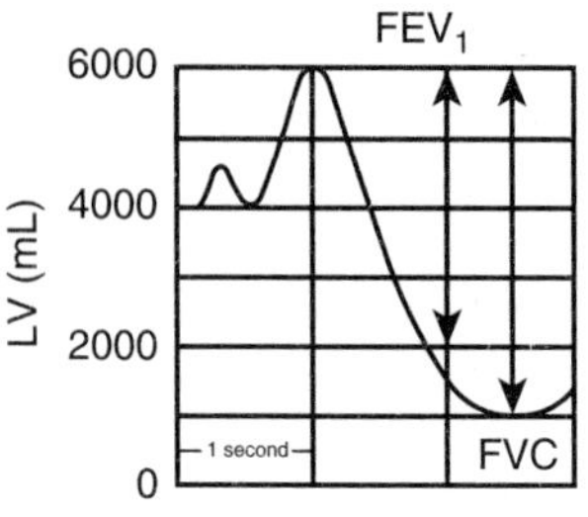 Spirometry pattern normal	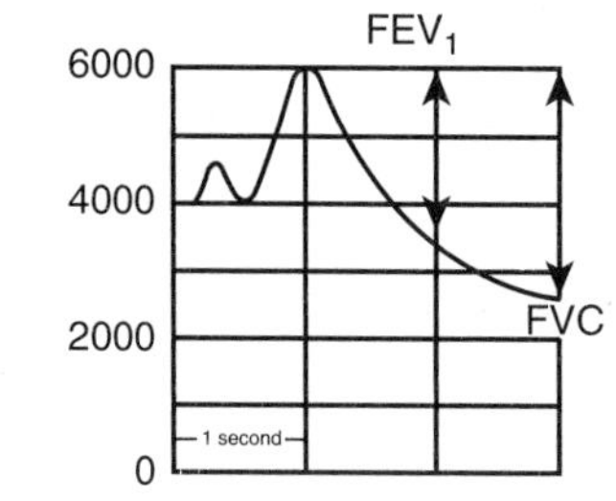 During a maximal forced expiration, a smaller than normal volume of air is expired more slowly	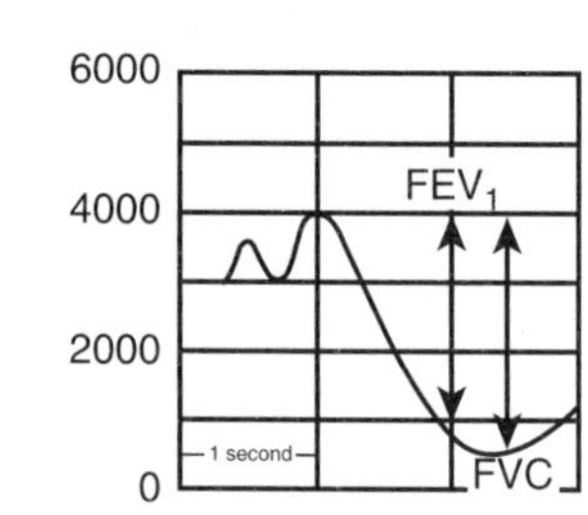 During a maximal forced expiration, a smaller than normal volume of air is expired more quickly and completely
Airway resistance normal	Airway resistance ↑	Airway resistance normal
Elastance normal	Elastance ↓	Elastance ↑
Compliance normal	Compliance ↑	Compliance ↓ Lungs are "stiff"
RV = 1200mL FRC = 2700mL TLC = 6700mL	RV = ↑ FRC = ↑ TLC = ↑ } Causes a "barrel chest" or expiring with "pursed lips"	RV = ↓ FRC = ↓ TLC = ↓
FEV$_1$ = 4400mL	FEV$_1$ = 2500mL (↓↓)	FEV$_1$ = 3200mL (↓)
FVC = 5500mL	FVC = 3500mL (↓)	FVC = 3400mL (↓)
$\dfrac{FEV_1}{FVC} = \dfrac{4400}{5500} = 0.8$ *	$\dfrac{FEV_1}{FVC} = \dfrac{2500}{3500} < 0.8$	$\dfrac{FEV_1}{FVC} = \dfrac{3200}{3400} > 0.8$
$\dot{V}_A / \dot{Q} = 0.8$	$\dot{V}_A / \dot{Q} = ↓$	$\dot{V}_A / \dot{Q} = ↓$
A – a gradient = 5	A – a gradient = ↑	A – a gradient = ↑
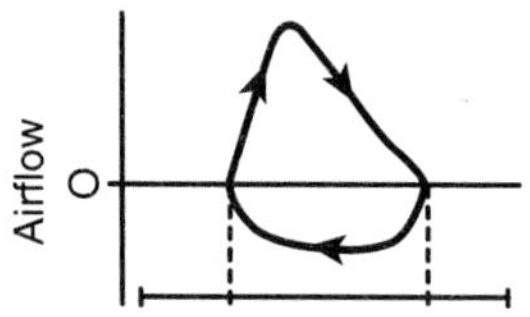 Volume Flow-volume curve	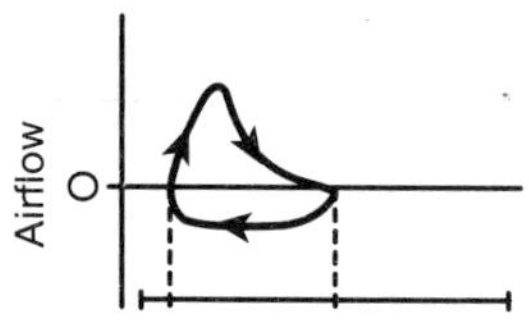 Volume Flow-volume curve Shifted to left	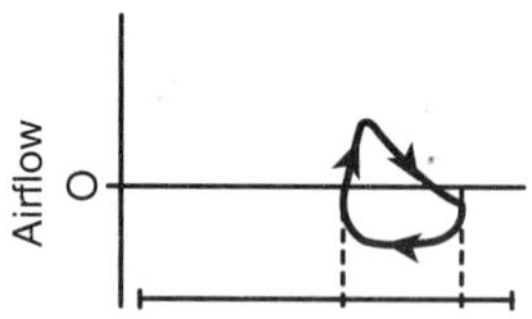 Volume Flow-volume curve Shifted to right

* In both obstructive and restrictive lung disease, FEV$_1$ and FVC are reduced (↓). However, in obstructive disease, FEV$_1$ is more dramatically reduced (↓↓) that results in a $\dfrac{FEV_1}{FVC}$ ratio < 0.8.

FIGURE 6-1. Comparison of various lung parameters in normal lung, obstructive lung disease (asthma, emphysema, chronic bronchitis), and restrictive lung disease (idiopathic pulmonary fibrosis). *Shaded blocks* indicate the hallmark signs of obstructive versus restrictive lung disease. FEV$_1$—forced expiratory volume; FRC—functional residual capacity; FVC—forced vital capacity; LV—lung volume; RV—residual volume; TLC—total lung capacity.

C. **Small cell carcinoma (SC)** has a 20% incidence and is associated with a **smoking history.** SC is centrally located, as it arises from larger bronchi. SC forms large, soft, gray–white masses and contains small, oval-shaped cells ("oat cells") derived from **Kulchitsky cells** (neural crest origin) that may produce **adrenocorticotropic hormone (ACTH)** or **antidiuretic hormone (ADH),** causing Cushing syndrome or syndrome of inappropriate secretion of ADH (SIADH), respectively. SC is a highly malignant and aggressive tumor (median survival time less than 3 months); however, these tumors do respond favorably to chemotherapy. Consequently, from the viewpoint of an oncologist there are two types of lung carcinomas: small cell carcinomas (chemotherapy-sensitive) and non-small cell carcinomas (chemotherapy nonsensitive).

D. **Undifferentiated large cell carcinoma (LC)** has a 10% incidence. LC is a diagnosis of exclusion in a poorly differentiated non-small cell carcinoma that does not show clear histological signs of either adenocarcinoma or squamous cell carcinoma.

E. **Carcinoid tumor (CT)** has a 2% incidence and is not associated with a smoking history. CT is a neuroendocrine neoplasm similar to Kulchitsky cells derived from the pluripotential basal layer of the respiratory epithelium. CT is generally endocrinologically silent. CT may be located centrally, peripherally, or in the midportion of the lung. Centrally located CT has a large endobronchial component with a smooth, fleshy mass protruding into the lumen of the bronchus. Patients with CT may develop **carcinoid syndrome,** which is characterized by: facial flushing (as a result of vasomotor disturbances), diarrhea (as a result of intestinal hypermotility), or wheezing (as a result of bronchoconstriction).

ⒾⓍ Cystic Fibrosis

Cystic fibrosis is caused by production of abnormally thick mucus by epithelial cells lining the respiratory (and gastrointestinal) tract. This results clinically in obstruction of airways and recurrent bacterial infections (e.g., *Staphylococcus aureus, Pseudomonas aeruginosa*). CF is caused by autosomal recessive mutations of the CF gene, which is located on the long arm of chromosome 7 (q7). The CF gene encodes for a protein called **CFTR** (**c**ystic **f**ibrosis **tr**ansporter), which functions as a **Cl$^-$ ion channel.** In North America, 70% of CF cases are due to a three-base deletion, which codes for the amino acid **phenylalanine at position #508** such that phenylalanine is missing from CFTR. Clinical signs include: meconium ileus (i.e., obstruction of the bowel) in the neonate, steatorrhea (fatty stool) or obstruction of the bowel in childhood, and **cor pulmonale** (manifesting as right-side heart failure) developing secondary to pulmonary hypertension.

Ⓧ Selected Photographs, Radiographs, and Micrographs

A. **Atelectasis, neonatal respiratory distress syndrome (NRDS), adult respiratory distress syndrome (ARDS), pulmonary infarction, pulmonary embolism, and bronchiectasis** *(Fig. 6-2)*

B. **Obstructive lung disease, asthma, emphysema, chronic bronchitis** *(Fig. 6-3)*

C. **Restrictive lung disease, idiopathic pulmonary fibrosis, coal workers pneumoconiosis (CWP), silicosis, asbestosis, and sarcoidosis** *(Fig. 6-4)*

D. **Cystic fibrosis** *(Fig. 6-5)*

E. **Bronchogenic carcinoma, adenocarcinoma subtypes, squamous cell carcinoma, small cell carcinoma, undifferentiated large cell carcinoma, and carcinoid tumor** *(Fig. 6-6)*

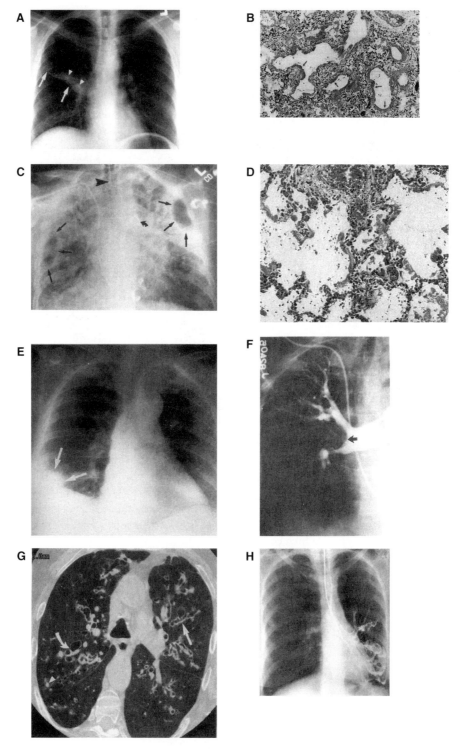

FIGURE 6-2. (A) Right upper lobe segmental atelectasis. PA radiograph shows partial collapse of the right upper lobe. The minor fissure is mildly elevated (*arrows*) outlining the lower border of the atelectatic lung. Note the calcified densities (*arrowheads*). **(B) LM of neonatal respiratory distress syndrome (NRDS).** The air-filled bronchioles and alveolar ducts are widely dilated. In addition, they are lined by a homogeneous hyaline membrane material (*arrows*) that consists of fibrin and necrotic cells. Note the atelectasis. **(C and D) Adult respiratory distress syndrome (ARDS). (C)** AP recumbent radiograph shows an endotracheal tube (*arrowhead*), oval collections of air at the periphery of the lung representing pneumatoceles (*arrows*), and a right subclavian Swan-Ganz catheter (*curved arrow*). **(D)** LM of ARDS. Note the patchy atelectasis, edema, hyaline membranes, and cellular debris in the alveoli. **(E) Pulmonary infarct.** PA radiograph shows a pleural-based, rounded area at the right costophrenic angle (Hampton hump), indicating an acute pulmonary infarct. **(F) Pulmonary embolism.** A pulmonary arteriogram shows a large saddle embolus (*arrow*). Note the poor perfusion of the right middle and lower lobes compared with the upper lobe. **(G and H) Bronchiectasis. (G)** High-resolution CT scan shows a beaded appearance of some airways called varicose bronchiectasis (*straight arrow*) and a cluster-of-grapes appearance of some airways called cystic bronchiectasis (*curved arrow*). The bronchial and bronchiolar walls are thickened, and some are filled with mucus-forming nodular opacities (*arrowhead*). **(H) Bronchogram.** The dilated bronchi have a saccular appearance and are clearly seen within the left lower lobe.

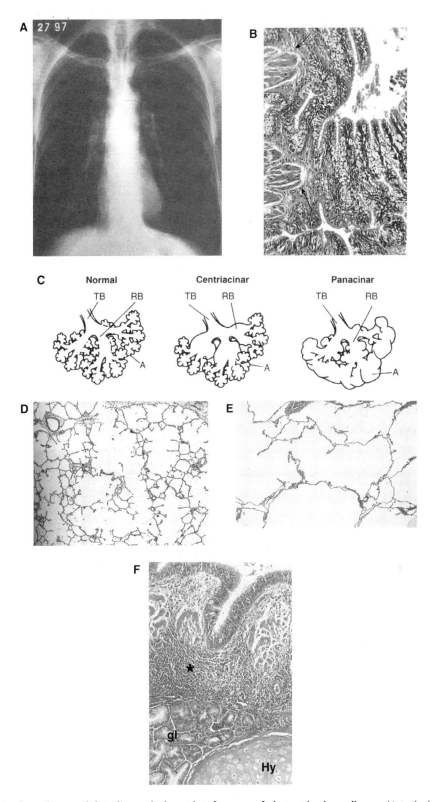

FIGURE 6-3. Obstructive lung disease. (A) Radiograph shows key features of obstructive lung disease. Note the hyperinflation of the lung and destruction of the lung interstitium (i.e., bulla formation) cause the lung to appear hyperlucent. Note that the diaphragm is flat and depressed (i.e., lower than rib 11). **(B) Asthma.** LM shows the respiratory epithelium that lines the bronchus forms invaginations and contains enlarged goblet cells that secrete mucus. Note the hyperplasia of bronchial smooth muscle (*arrows*). **(C–E) Emphysema. (C)** Diagram shows a normal pulmonary lobule, centriacinar emphysema, and panacinar emphysema. In the normal, the terminal bronchiole (*TB*), respiratory bronchiole (*RB*), and alveoli (*A*) are normal size. In centriacinar emphysema, the respiratory bronchioles only are enlarged. In panacinar emphysema, the alveolar ducts, alveolar sacs, and alveoli are all enlarged. **(D)** LM shows the histological appearance of normal lung parenchyma. **(E)** LM shows the histological appearance of panacinar emphysema with large, irregular airspaces and reduced number of alveolar walls. **(F) Chronic bronchitis.** LM shows the wall of the bronchus contains a large number of inflammatory cells (*) and hypertrophy of seromucous glands (*gl*). HY—hyaline cartilage.

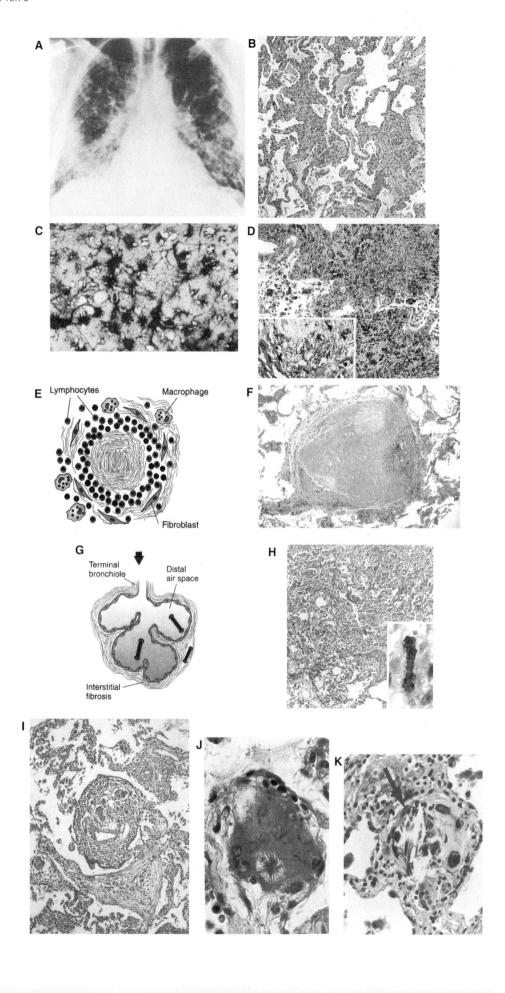

FIGURE 6-4. Restrictive lung disease. (A) Radiograph shows key features of restrictive lung disease. Note a reticular pattern of lung opacities, as a result of an abnormal lung interstitium, that are interspersed between clear areas (lung cysts or "honeycomb lung"), small, contracted lung, and raised diaphragm. **(B) Idiopathic pulmonary fibrosis (IPF).** LM shows the appearance of usual interstitial pneumonia, which is the most common form of IPF. Note the inflammatory cell infiltrates with the interalveolar septae, thickened interalveolar septae resulting from fibrosis, and fibrin in the alveolar spaces**. (C and D) Coal worker's pneumoconiosis (CWP). (C)** Photograph of a gross specimen of a coal miner's lung showing scattered, irregular, carbon-pigmented nodules throughout the lung parenchyma. **(D)** LM shows fibrotic carbon-pigmented nodules. Inset shows numerous silica particles that appear as birefringent crystals under polarized light. **(E and F) Silicosis. (E)** Diagram of a silicotic nodule. In silicosis, the silica particles are toxic to alveolar macrophages, which die and release fibrogenic factors that produce small, dense, collagenous nodules. **(F)** LM of a silicotic nodule shows whorls of dense collagen fibers. **(G and H) Asbestosis. (G)** Diagram of asbestosis. In asbestosis, there is prominent diffuse pulmonary interstitial fibrosis and asbestos bodies. **(H)** LM shows prominent diffuse pulmonary interstitial fibrosis and an asbestos body (*inset*). **(I–K) Sarcoidosis. (I)** LM shows a noncaseating granuloma characteristic of sarcoidosis containing epithelioid cells, Langerhans cells, and giant cells. **(J)** LM shows a stellate inclusion body within a giant cell called an asteroid body. **(K)** LM shows a laminated concretion of calcium and proteins (*arrow*) called a Schaumann body.

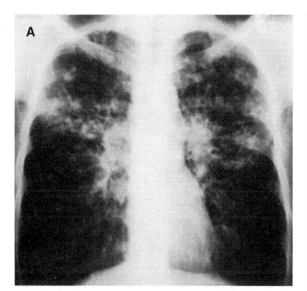

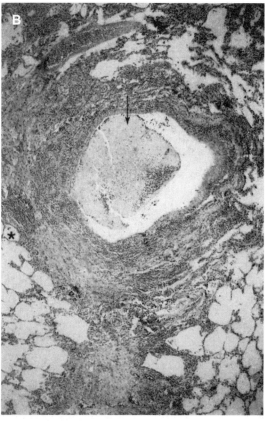

FIGURE 6-5. Cystic fibrosis. (A) PA radiograph of cystic fibrosis shows hyperinflation of both lungs, reduced size of the heart as a result of pulmonary compression, cyst formation, and atelectasis (collapse of alveoli) in both lungs. **(B)** LM of cystic fibrosis shows a bronchus that is filled with thick mucus and inflammatory cells (*arrow*). Smaller bronchi may be completely plugged by this material. In addition, surrounding the bronchus there is heavy lymphocyte infiltration (*).

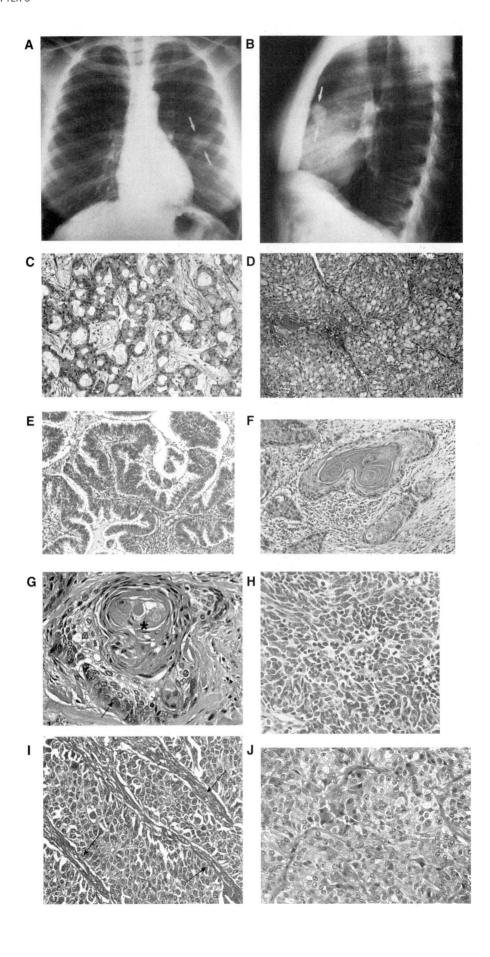

FIGURE 6-6. (A and B) Bronchogenic carcinoma. (A) PA radiograph shows a 3-cm nodule in the left lung (*arrows*). **(B)** Lateral radiograph shows the nodule (*arrows*) anterior within the left upper lobe. **(C) LM of adenocarcinoma acinar subtype.** Note the cuboidal- or polygonal-shaped cells containing mucus arranged in an acinus resembling the normal seromucous glands present within bronchi. **(D) LM of adenocarcinoma solid with mucus formation subtype.** Note the cuboidal- or polygonal-shaped cells containing mucus arranged in solid cell nests (i.e., no glandular formation). The individual cells may demonstrate a signet-ring form similar to normal adipocytes. These tumors may be immunocytochemically positive for lactoferrin. **(E) LM of adenocarcinoma papillary subtype.** Note the tall, columnar-shaped cells (no cilia are present) arranged in a papillary fashion on a distinctive core of fibrovascular connective tissue. **(F) LM of adenocarcinoma bronchioloalveolar subtype.** Note the tall, columnar-shaped cells containing mucus and lining the alveoli by replacing the squamous type I pneumocytes normally present. This is a mucinous bronchioloalveolar subtype. **(G) LM of squamous cell carcinoma.** Note the polygonal-shaped cells arranged in solid cell nests (*arrow*) and bright eosinophilic aggregates of extracellular keratin (*). Intracellular keratinization may also be apparent such that the cytoplasm appears glassy and eosinophilic. In well-differentiated squamous cell carcinomas, intercellular bridges may be observed, which are cytoplasmic extensions between adjacent cells. Another important histological characteristic of squamous cell carcinoma is the in situ replacement of the bronchial epithelium. As a rule, neither adenocarcinoma nor small cell carcinoma replaces the bronchial epithelium, but instead, tends to grow beneath the epithelium. **(H) LM of small cell carcinoma.** Note the small, oval-shaped cells arranged in sheets with hyperchromatic nuclei, no nucleoli, scanty cytoplasm, and ill-defined cell borders. By electron microscopy, neurosecretory granules can be observed. **(I) LM of undifferentiated large cell carcinoma.** Not the large, polygonal-shaped cells arranged in solid cell nests with vesicular nuclei, prominent nucleoli, moderately abundant cytoplasm, and well-defined cell borders. Note the distinctive fibrovascular connective tissue (*arrows*). **(J) LM of carcinoid tumor.** Note the polygonal-shaped cells arranged in solid cell nests with uniform nuclei demonstrating a finely granular chromatin pattern and a light eosinophilic to clear cytoplasm. By electron microscopy, neurosecretory granules can be observed

◀

Chapter 7

Microbiology

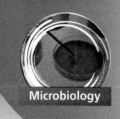

Microbiology

❶ Bacterial Pneumonia

Pneumonia is a general term that describes exudative inflammation and consolidation (solidification) of the lung parenchyma. Traditionally, pneumonias were classified as **bronchopneumonia** (characterized by patchy consolidation of the lung, frequently multilobar, bilateral, and basal because of gravitational pooling of bacteria) or **lobar pneumonia** (consolidation of an entire lobe), but with the effectiveness of modern antibiotics this classification is not clinically relevant today.

A. Pneumococcal pneumonia

1. **General features.** *Streptococcus pneumoniae* causes pneumococcal pneumonia. Pneumococcal pneumonia is the **most common bacterial pneumonia in older adults (>65 years of age).** Pneumococcal pneumonia is generally a consequence of altered immunity within the respiratory tract most frequently following a viral infection (e.g., influenza), which damages the mucociliary elevator, or chronic obstructive pulmonary disease (COPD), or alcoholism. Four stages of a classic bacterial pneumonia are described: 1) The **initial stage** features acute congestion, intra-alveolar fluid containing many bacteria, and few neutrophils. 2) The **early consolidation** or **"red hepatization"** (2–4 days) stage features consolidation with infiltration of large numbers of neutrophils and intra-alveolar hemorrhage. The lung is red as a result of extravasated RBCs, firm and airless with a liver-like consistency. 3) The **late consolidation** or **"gray hepatization"** (4–8 days) stage features large amounts of fibrin within the alveoli, lysis of the neutrophils, and appearance of macrophages, which phagocytose the inflammatory debris. The lung has a gray-brown dry surface. 4) The **resolution** stage begins after 8 days. Clinical findings include acute onset with fever, chills, chest pain secondary to pleural involvement, and hemoptysis (rusty, blood-tinged sputum).

   [handwritten marginal note:] red – 2-4 gray 4-8

2. **Causative agent (*Streptococcus pneumoniae*).** The genus *Streptococcus* are **Gram-positive cocci** that are arranged in pairs or chains, all of which are Gram-positive cocci, facultative anaerobic, and catalase-negative. *Streptococcus pneumoniae* is Gram-positive, facultative anaerobic, catalase-negative, α-hemolytic (a greenish zone surrounding a bacterial colony grown on blood-agar medium), lancet-shaped diplococcus whose growth is inhibited by Optochin and lysed by bile.

3. **Identification.** The Lancefield extraction method and capillary precipitin test are the time-honored techniques for the identification of the groupable streptococci. *Streptococcus pneumonia* is typed using capsular antibodies and may be identified by the quellung reaction (capsular swelling). Gram stain of CSF sediment and capsular antigen tests are the rapid diagnostic tests for meningitis.

4. **Reservoir.** *Streptococcus pneumonia* normally colonizes the nasopharyngeal mucosa and may reach the lungs if the cough reflex is suppressed (e.g., alcoholics) or if the mucociliary elevator is damaged.

5. **Virulence factors.** *Streptococcus pneumonia* has a **capsule** that is resistant to phagocytosis by alveolar macrophages until opsonized; produces **pneumolysin O,** which damages respiratory epithelium by binding to the host cell membrane and creating pores; produces secretory IgA protease; and stimulates fluid, RBCs, and inflammatory cell movement into the alveolar airspace. Asplenic patients are routinely vaccinated with pneumococcal vaccine, which contains 23 different capsular serotypes.

6. **Other diseases**
    a. **Meningitis in adults** is most commonly caused by *Streptococcus pneumoniae,* whereby peptidoglycan/teichoic acid triggers an inflammatory response in the central nervous system resulting in elevated cell counts in the cerebrospinal fluid.
    b. **Otitis media** is most commonly caused by *Streptococcus pneumoniae.*

B. **Streptococcal pneumonia**
    1. **General features.** *Streptococcus pyogenes* causes streptococcal pneumonia. Streptococcal pneumonia is generally uncommon in the community. However, it may have been the superinfection in the 1918–1919 influenza pandemic and is seen in chronically ill patients. The late consolidation stage or "gray hepatization" stage (as seen in pneumococcal pneumonia; see above) is absent (i.e., the lungs of patients who die of streptococcal pneumonia are heavy and show bloody edema). The alveoli are filled with large amounts of fibrin but few neutrophils. Clinical findings include: abrupt fever, cough, dyspnea, chest pain, hemoptysis, and often cyanosis.
    2. **Causative agent (*Streptococcus pyogenes*; group A streptococcus).** The genus *Streptococcus* are **Gram-positive cocci** that are arranged in pairs or chains, all of which are Gram-positive cocci, facultative anaerobic, and catalase-negative. *Streptococcus pyogenes* (group A streptococcus) is Gram-positive, facultative anaerobe, catalase-negative, β-hemolytic, bacitracin-sensitive, and occurs in chains.
    3. **Identification.** For pharyngitis: a rapid antigen test is used (if negative, proceed to culture). In a person with repeated positive throat cultures, negative ASO titers suggest a pharyngeal carrier state. For invasive disease: culture is used. For rheumatic fever: ASO titers >200 are positive.
    4. **Reservoir.** *Streptococcus pyogenes* normally colonizes the oropharyngeal mucosa of human carriers.
    5. **Virulence factors.** *Streptococcus pyogenes* has a **hyaluronic acid capsule** that is resistant to phagocytosis; expresses **M proteins** on the cell surface that convey antigenic variability observed among 80 different serotypes of M proteins; produces **streptolysin O** (oxygen-labile hemolysin), which lyses RBCs, leukocytes, and platelets; streptolysin O is highly immunogenic and anti-streptolysin O is readily produced, which is the basis of the **ASO test**; produces **C5a peptidase**, which degrades C5a that recruits and activates phagocytic cells; produces *Streptococcal pyogenes* **erythrogenic toxins (SPE A-C)**, which are phage-coded superantigens, which activate T cells and macrophages to release cytokines and reduce normal liver clearance of endogenous endotoxin.
    6. **Other diseases.** *Streptococcus pyogenes* is responsible for other diseases, some of which are much more common clinically.
        a. **"Strep throat"** presents as pharyngitis with tonsillar exudate, anterior cervical lymphadenopathy, fever, and nausea.
        b. **Scarlatina** (if mild) or **scarlet fever** (if severe) is "strep throat" with a rash and involves SPE A-C erythrogenic toxins.
        c. **Streptococcal impetigo** is characterized by golden-crusted skin lesions.
        d. **Necrotizing fasciitis** is the collective effect of *Streptococcal pyogenes'* virulence factors that cause a rapid, life-threatening infection.
        e. **Poststreptococcal sequelae. Acute glomerulonephritis** presents as hypertension, edema, and dark urine as a result of hematuria or proteinuria. It is usually an M12 serotype and a sequelae to pharyngitis or impetigo. **Rheumatic fever** presents with fever, carditis, subcutaneous nodules, polyarthritis, and chorea. It is a sequelae to untreated *Streptococcal pyogenes* pharyngitis.

PSGN - M12

C. **Streptococcal pneumonia in the newborn**
    1. **General features.** *Streptococcus agalactiae* causes streptococcal pneumonia in the newborn. Streptococcal pneumonia in the newborn produces symptoms similar to

infantile respiratory distress syndrome. However, the infants are full term, develop severe toxemia, and may die within a few hours. The **early onset (1–7 days)** is characterized by respiratory problems, sepsis, pneumonia, and meningitis. The **late onset** is characterized by septicemia and meningitis. The incidence of streptococcal pneumonia in the newborn can be reduced by penicillin administration to pregnant women with the following conditions: fever of unknown origin, *Streptococcus agalactiae* urinary tract infection (UTI), delivery <37 weeks, or amniochorionic membrane rupture >18 hours.

2. **Causative agent (*Streptococcus agalactiae;* group B streptococcus).** The genus ***Streptococcus*** are **Gram-positive cocci** that are arranged in pairs or chains, all of which are Gram-positive cocci, facultative anaerobic, and catalase-negative. *Streptococcus agalactiae* (group B streptococcus) is Gram-positive, facultative anaerobic, catalase-negative, β-hemolytic, bacitracin-resistant, and occurs in chains.

3. **Reservoir.** *Streptococcus agalactiae* normally colonizes the genitourinary (GU) tract and gastrointestinal (GI) tract.

4. **Virulence factors.** *Streptococcus agalactiae* has a **polysaccharide capsule** that is resistant to phagocytosis.

5. **Other diseases.** In adults, *Streptococcus agalactiae* may cause symptomatic fever and urinary tract infections (UTIs) in pregnant women, leading to amnionitis or endometritis.

D. Staphylococcal pneumonia

1. **General features.** *Staphylococcus aureus* cause staphylococcal pneumonia. Staphylococcal pneumonia is generally uncommon in the community. However, it is prevalent as a superinfection after influenza or viral infections of the respiratory tract, in intubated patients and cystic fibrosis patients, and as a nosocomial infection in chronically ill patients. Staphylococcal pneumonia is characterized by **many small lung abscesses,** which may lead to **pneumatoceles** (a thin-walled cystic space) that rupture into the pleural cavity and cause tension pneumothorax.

2. **Causative agent (*Staphylococcus aureus*).** The genus ***Staphylococcus*** is **Gram-positive cocci** that tend to grow in clusters and are catalase-positive. *Staphylococcus aureus* is Gram-positive, aerobic or facultative anaerobic, catalase-positive, coagulase-positive (initiates the formation of a fibrin clot), β-hemolytic (a clear zone surrounding a bacterial colony grown on blood-agar medium), salt tolerant (halodermic), contains protein A (binds to Fc fragment of IgG and inhibits phagocytosis), produces a yellow pigment, and may produce exotoxins.

3. **Identification.** *Staphylococcus aureus* is identified as a Gram-positive staphylococcus that is catalase-positive, coagulase-positive. The screening medium is mannitol-salt medium.

4. **Reservoir.** *Staphylococcus aureus* normally colonizes the nasopharyngeal mucosa and resides on the skin. *Staphylococcus aureus* is transmitted by sneezing, skin lesions, and touch with the hands.

5. **Drug resistance.** Methicillin-resistant *Staphylococcus aureus* (MRSA) is due to the acquisition of the ***mecA* gene** that codes for an abnormal **penicillin-binding protein (PBP2′)** that does not bind penicillins. Expression of PBP2′ renders bacteria resistant to all β-lactam antibiotics (including cephalosporins and carbapenems). Most MRSA strains also have plasmid-mediated resistance to other drugs except glycopeptides (e.g., vancomycin).

6. **Virulence factors.** *Staphylococcus aureus* contains **protein A** on the cell surface that binds the F_c portion of IgG and prevents antibody-mediated clearance of the bacteria. *Staphylococcus aureus* produces **five cytolytic toxins (α, β, Δ, γ, Panton-Valentine leukocidin). α toxin** is a 33,000d protein that integrates into the host cell membrane (e.g., RBCs, leukocytes, hepatocytes, platelets, and smooth muscle cells), forming 1–2-nm pores that lead to osmotic swelling and cell lysis. **β toxin (sphingomyelinase C)** is a 35,000d protein that catalyzes the hydrolysis of phospholipids in the host cell membrane (e.g., RBCs, leukocytes, macrophages, and

fibroblasts) proportional to the amount of sphingomyelin exposed on the cell surface. **Δ toxin** is a 3,000d polypeptide that disrupts the cell membrane and intracellular membranes by a detergent-like action. **γ toxin and Panton-Valentine leukocidin** are bicomponent toxins [composed of two polypeptide chains: the S (slow-eluting) component and the F (fast-eluting) component] that integrate into the host cell membrane (e.g., RBCs, neutrophils, macrophages), forming 1–2-nm pores that lead to osmotic swelling and cell lysis. *Staphylococcus aureus* produces two exfoliative toxins (ETA and ETB). **ETA** is a heat-stable serine protease whose gene is chromosomal. **ETB** is a heat-labile serine protease and is plasmid-mediated. ETA and ETB promote the splitting of desmosomes within the stratum granulosum of the skin epidermis. *Staphylococcus aureus* produces **eight enterotoxins (A–E, G–I).** All the enterotoxins are heat-stable (heating to 100°C for 30 minutes) and hydrolysis-resistant to gastric and jejunal enzymes. The precise mechanism of action is not known; however, these enterotoxins are superantigens, which activate T cells causing release of cytokines and mast cells causing release of inflammatory mediators. *Staphylococcus aureus* produces **toxic shock syndrome toxin-1 (TSST-1). TSST-1** is a 22,000d heat-stable, proteolysis-resistant protein whose gene is chromosomal. TSST-1 is a superantigen, which activates T cells and macrophages causing release of cytokines and which reduces normal liver clearance of endogenous endotoxin.

7. **Other diseases.** *Staphylococcus aureus* is responsible for other diseases, some of which are much more common clinically.

   a. ***Staphylococcus aureus* food poisoning** presents as rapid onset (1–6 hours) of abdominal pain, vomiting, and diarrhea caused by heat-stable enterotoxins (A–E, G–I) produced in poorly refrigerated, *Staphylococcus aureus*-contaminated foods.

   b. ***Staphylococcus aureus* skin or subcutaneous infections** present as subcutaneous tenderness and heat, redness, and swelling with a surgery or neutropenia predisposition. This infection may lead to **scalded skin syndrome** if exfoliative toxins ETA and ETB are produced. **Staphylococcal impetigo** is characterized by large bullae (vesicles).

   c. **Toxic shock syndrome (TSS)** presents as fever, hypotension, scarlatiniform rash, desquamation of palms and soles, multiorgan failure with surgical packing or super tampon use predisposition. TSST-1 plays a prominent role.

   d. **Acute endocarditis** presents as fever, malaise, leukocytosis, and heart murmur caused by cytolytic toxins (α, β, Δ, γ, Panton-Valentine leukocidin), which rapidly damage the heart. Acute endocarditis is most commonly caused by *Staphylococcus aureus*.

E. *Klebsiella* pneumonia

   1. **General features.** *Klebsiella pneumoniae* causes *Klebsiella* pneumonia. The stages of *Klebsiella* pneumonia are not as well described as those of pneumococcal pneumonia (see above), with the level of congestion and hemorrhage less pronounced. *Klebsiella* pneumonia is characterized by an increased size of the affected lobe so that the fissure bulges in the direction of the normal region of the lung. *Klebsiella* pneumonia may be associated with necrosis, abscess formation, and a **bronchopleural fistula** (an abnormal communication between the bronchial airway and pleural cavity). Clinical findings include: onset is less dramatic than pneumococcal pneumonia, occurs in patients with underlying pulmonary disease or alcoholism, dark-red, bloody nonmalodorous sputum (currant jelly sputum), and produces difficult-to-treat abscesses.

   2. **Causative agent (*Klebsiella pneumoniae*).** The genus ***Klebsiella*** belonging to the **Enterobacteriaceae family** are **Gram-negative facultative anaerobic bacilli,** all of which are Gram-negative rods, facultative anaerobic, catalase-positive, oxidase-negative, ferment glucose, and reduced nitrites to nitrates. *Klebsiella pneumoniae* is a lactose-fermenting rod.

3. **Reservoir.** *Klebsiella pneumoniae* normally colonizes the upper respiratory tract and GI tract and is generally an opportunistic infection.
4. **Virulence factors.** *Klebsiella pneumoniae* has a thick, gelatinous, polysaccharide capsule.

F. **Other pneumonias.** There are opportunistic pneumonias that are caused by Gram-negative bacteria, which include *Escherichia coli, Pseudomonas aeruginosa, and Haemophilus influenza.*

Ⅱ Viral and Mycoplasma Pneumonia

This type of pneumonia (in contrast with bacterial pneumonia; see IA) is characterized by patchy inflammation confined predominately to the interalveolar septae and pulmonary interstitium. The affected areas of the lung are red–blue, congested, and subcrepitant. This type of pneumonia is also called **primary atypical pneumonia** or **interstitial pneumonitis.** The word "atypical" refers to the lack of an intra-alveolar exudate that is so prominent in a bacterial pneumonia. Four stages of interstitial pneumonitis are described: 1) the **initial stage** features entry of the infectious agent into the alveoli by inhalation; 2) the **necrosis stage** features infection and necrosis of type I pneumocytes, which results in the formation of hyaline membranes; 3) the **hyperplasia stage** features hyperplasia of type II pneumocytes followed by inflammation of the interalveolar septae and pulmonary interstitium that is characterized by mononuclear inflammatory cells (i.e., lymphocytes, macrophages, and plasma cells), edema, and congested capillaries; and 4) the **resolution stage.** Note that interstitial pneumonitis is characterized by inflammation within the interalveolar septae and pulmonary interstitium; whereas, bacterial pneumonia is characterized by inflammation within the alveoli.

A. **Cytomegalovirus (CMV) pneumonia**
1. **General features.** CMV causes a pneumonia showing **interstitial pneumonitis** initially described in infants but now prevalent in immunocompromised patients. CMV infection is characterized by enlarged cells (i.e., cytomegalic cells), which contain a dense, central, nuclear inclusion body with a peripheral halo (**owl's-eye appearance**).
2. **Causative agent (cytomegalovirus).** Cytomegalovirus belonging to the **Herpesvirus family** is a **linear, double-stranded DNA virus.** The virion is an **enveloped** (with the host cell nuclear membrane) 150-nm diameter **icosahedron.** The capsid consists of 162 capsomeres. The **tegument** is the space between the envelope and capsid and contains viral proteins and enzymes that initiate viral replication.
3. **Replication**
    a. **Infection and entry.** As herpes viruses in general, CMV infects the host cell through viral glycoproteins on the viral envelope binding to host cell receptors, causing a fusion of the viral envelope and host cell membrane. The nucleocapsid enters the host cell cytoplasm, viral proteins and enzymes from the tegument enter the cytoplasm, and the capsid delivers the viral DNA into the host cell nucleus.
    b. **Early transcriptional events.** These include synthesis of transcription factors, various enzymes, and DNA polymerase.
    c. **Replication of the viral genome.** Viral DNA replication occurs in the host cell nucleus and is mediated by viral DNA polymerase. Viral enzymes provide deoxyribonucleotide substrates for the viral DNA polymerase, and these enzymes are the targets of many antiviral drugs.
    d. **Viral assembly.** Late transcriptional events include the synthesis of capsid proteins in the host cell cytoplasm, which are then transported to the host cell nucleus for viral assembly. CMV is enveloped with the host cell nuclear membrane.

   e.   **Viral release.** CMV is released by lysis of the host cell or budding from the host cell after passing through the Golgi.
4. **Identification.** CMV can be grown in diploid fibroblast cell cultures that are cultured for 4–6 weeks. Monoclonal antibodies, DNA probes, and the polymerase chain reaction (PCR) can detect CMV antigens or the CMV genome. Seroconversion (CMV-specific IgM antibodies) is an excellent marker for primary infections. CMV infection can be identified by the histological observation of cytomegalic cells (owl's-eye appearance) stained with Papanicolaou or hematoxylin-eosin stains.
5. **Reservoir.** CMV is a common human pathogen present in approximately 50% of adults in developed countries and in 1 to 2.5% of newborns. CMV can be isolated from urine, feces, blood, throat washings, saliva, tears, organs for transplantation, semen, amniotic fluid, breast milk, vaginal secretions, and cervical secretions. CMV is an opportunistic infection in immunocompromised patients and rarely causes symptoms in the immunocompetent person. In adults, CMV is transmitted most commonly by blood transfusion, organ transplantation, and sexual contact. In fetuses, CMV is transmitted transplacentally and by CMV ascending from the cervix during a recurrence. In perinates, CMV is transmitted during passage through the birth canal and through breast milk. CMV establishes a **latent infection in lymphocytes, stromal cells of the bone marrow,** and other cells.
6. **Other diseases.** CMV is a ubiquitous virus and is the **most common fetal infection.** CMV is transmitted to the fetus **transplacentally** or by **CMV ascending from the cervix during a recurrence** with more severe malformations when infection occurs during the first half of pregnancy. CMV is also transmitted to perinates during passage through the birth canal or through breast milk, but causes no apparent disease. Both primary and recurrent infections of the mother can result in transmission of CMV to the fetus. In mothers with recurrent infection, the presence of CMV antibodies does not prevent CMV transmission to the fetus but does protect the fetus from major fetal malformations. Consequently, the risk of major fetal malformations is much higher in infants of mothers who had a primary CMV infection during pregnancy compared to mothers who have had recurrent infections. The most common manifestation of CMV fetal infection is **sensorineural deafness. Cytomegalic inclusion disease** (characterized by multiorgan involvement) is the most serious but least common manifestation of CMV infection and results in: intrauterine growth retardation, microcephaly, chorioretinitis, hepatosplenomegaly, osteitis (celery stalk appearance of long bones), discrete cerebral calcifications, mental retardation, heart block, and bluish-purple lesions on a yellow jaundiced skin ("blueberry muffin spots"). Ganciclovir treatment of the neonate is being evaluated for symptomatic congenital CMV infection.

B. Varicella (VZV) pneumonia
1. **General features.** VZV causes disseminated, focally necrotic lesions in the lung that may escalate to a pneumonia showing an **interstitial pneumonitis.** VZV infection is characterized by cells (sometimes multinucleated) that contain an eosinophilic, refractile nuclear inclusion body with a peripheral halo (Cowdry type A).
2. **Causative agent (varicella-zoster virus; VZV).** VZV belonging to the **Herpesvirus family** is a **linear, double-stranded DNA virus.** The virion is an **enveloped** (with the host cell nuclear membrane), 150-nm diameter **icosahedron.** The capsid consists of capsomeres. The **tegument** is the space between the envelope and capsid and contains viral proteins and enzymes that initiate viral replication.
3. **Replication.**
   a.   **Infection and entry.** As herpes viruses do in general, VZV infects the host cell through viral glycoproteins on the viral envelope binding to host cell receptors causing a fusion of the viral envelope and host cell membrane. The nucleocapsid enters the host cell cytoplasm, viral proteins and enzymes from the

tegument enter the cytoplasm, and the capsid delivers the viral DNA into the host cell nucleus.

b. **Early transcriptional events.** These include synthesis of transcription factors, various enzymes, and DNA polymerase.

c. **Replication of the viral genome.** Viral DNA replication occurs in the host cell nucleus and is mediated by viral DNA polymerase. Viral enzymes (e.g., **thymidine kinase**) provide deoxyribonucleotide substrates for the viral DNA polymerase, and these enzymes are the targets of many antiviral drugs.

d. **Viral assembly.** Late transcriptional events include the synthesis of capsid proteins in the host cell cytoplasm, which are then transported to the host cell nucleus for viral assembly. CMV is enveloped with the host cell nuclear membrane.

e. **Viral release.** VZV is released by lysis of the host cell or budding from the host cell after passing through the Golgi.

4. **Identification.** VZV is difficult to grow in diploid fibroblast cell cultures. Monoclonal antibodies and PCR can detect VZV membrane antigens and the VZV genome. A high titer of VZV antibody is observed in patients with a herpes zoster outbreak. VZV infection can be identified by histological observation of cells from vesicle scrapings, skin lesions, respiratory specimens, or organ biopsy specimens that show multinucleation (i.e., syncytia) and Cowdry type A inclusion bodies.

5. **Reservoir.** VZV is an extremely communicable human pathogen present in approximately 90% of adults in developed countries. VZV is an opportunistic infection in immunocompromised patients. VZV is transmitted by respiratory droplets and direct contact of the skin vesicles. Patients are contagious before and during the symptoms. VZV establishes a **latent infection** in neurons of the dorsal root or cranial nerve ganglia and results in **herpes zoster** upon reactivation.

6. **Other diseases**

a. **Varicella (chickenpox).** Varicella or chickenpox is one of the five classic childhood exanthems, which includes: rubella, roseola, measles, and fifth disease. Chickenpox results from a primary infection with VZV whose clinical findings include: fever and an asynchronous maculopapular rash (present on the scalp and most severely on the thorax) that appears after a 14-day incubation period. The maculopapular lesions form a thin-walled vesicle on erythematous base ("dewdrop on a rose petal") that are the hallmark of chickenpox. The vesicles develop into pustules and crust over (within 12 hours) while a new crop of lesions appears, after which scabs form.

b. **Herpes zoster (shingles).** Herpes zoster is the recurrence of a latent VZV infection whose clinical findings include: a chickenpox-like rash and severe pain in a thoracic dermatome supplied by the nerve whose neurons are latently infected with VZV.

c. **Fetal varicella syndrome.** VZV is transmitted to the fetus **transplacentally** in 25% of cases, but fetal varicella syndrome develops only when maternal VZV infection occurs in the first trimester. The clinical manifestations of fetal varicella syndrome include: cicatricial (scarring) skin lesions in a dermatomal pattern, limb and digit hypoplasia, limb paresis/paralysis, hydrocephalus, microcephaly/mental retardation, seizures, chorioretinitis, and cataracts. Neonates whose mothers develop chickenpox 6–21 days before delivery do not show signs of severe chickenpox because maternal antibodies are produced and delivered to the fetus. Neonates whose mothers develop chickenpox fewer than 5 days before delivery or 2 days postpartum develop severe chickenpox with increased mortality and morbidity (i.e., fever, skin lesions, hemorrhagic rash, respiratory distress, and pneumonia).

C. **Adenovirus pneumonia**

1. **General features.** Adenovirus causes **acute respiratory tract disease** (primarily in military recruits) whose clinical findings include: fever, cough, pharyngitis, and

cervical adenitis. Adenovirus may also cause **other respiratory tract diseases** whose clinical findings include: cold-like symptoms, laryngitis, croup, necrotizing bronchiolitis, and pertussis-like illness, which may escalate to a pneumonia showing an **interstitial pneumonitis.** Adenovirus infection is characterized by cells that contain both eosinophilic nuclear inclusion bodies (similar to herpes infections) and indistinct, basophilic nuclear inclusion bodies (called **smudge cells**).

2. **Causative agent (adenovirus).** Adenoviruses (42 different serotypes) belonging to the *Adenovirus* family are **linear, double-stranded DNA viruses** with **terminal proteins** located at the 5′ end. The virions are **naked** (nonenveloped), 70–90-nm diameter **icosahedrons.** The capsid consists of 252 capsomers with 240 hexons and 12 pentons. The 12 pentons are associated with **fibers** that serve as **viral attachment proteins (VAPs)** and also carry **type-specific antigens.**

3. **Replication**
   a. **Infection and entry.** Adenovirus infects the host cell through fiber VAPs binding to a host cell receptor called the **Coxsackie adenovirus receptor (CAR).** The adenovirus enters the host cell cytoplasm by receptor-mediated endocytosis, lyses the endolysosomes, and the capsid delivers the viral DNA into the host cell nucleus.
   b. **Early transcriptional events.** These include the synthesis of proteins that stimulate cell growth, proteins that suppress the host immune response, a protein that binds to class I MHC and prevents class I MHC from reaching the host cell membrane, a DNA polymerase, and short virus-associated RNA segments (va RNAs) that block enzymes of the interferon-induced antiviral state of the host cell.
   c. **Replication of viral genome.** Viral DNA replication occurs in the host cell nucleus and is mediated by viral DNA polymerase using the terminal protein as a primer.
   d. **Viral assembly.** Late transcriptional events include the synthesis of capsid proteins in the host cell cytoplasm, which are then transported to the host cell nucleus for viral assembly.
   e. **Viral release.** The adenovirus is released by lysis of the host cell.

4. **Identification.** Adenovirus can be grown in cell culture whereby viral infection causes lysis and characteristic nuclear inclusion bodies within 2–20 days.

5. **Reservoir.** Adenovirus is transmitted by respiratory droplets or fecal–oral contact promoted by close human contact (e.g., classrooms, day care centers, military barracks). Adenovirus is resistant to drying, detergents, GI secretion, and mild chlorine treatment. Serotypes 1–7 are the most prevalent.

6. **Other diseases**
   a. **Acute febrile pharyngitis and pharyngoconjunctival fever.** Adenovirus causes pharyngitis in young children (<3 years of age) whose clinical findings include: mild flu-like symptoms that may last 3–5 days. Adenovirus also causes pharyngoconjunctival fever ("pink eye") in older children.
   b. **Conjunctivitis.** Adenovirus causes a follicular conjunctivitis that is characterized by a pebbled palpebral conjunctiva and inflammation of both the palpebral and bulbar conjunctiva.
   c. **Acute viral gastroenteritis.** Adenovirus causes acute viral gastroenteritis. Serotypes 40–42 are grouped together as enteric adenoviruses and cause diarrhea in infants.

D. **Rubeola (measles) pneumonia**
   1. **General features.** Rubeola causes a pneumonia showing **interstitial pneumonitis.** Rubeola infection is characterized by large, multinucleated giant cells, which contain both an eosinophilic nuclear inclusion body and eosinophilic, irregular cytoplasmic inclusion bodies.
   2. **Causative agent (rubeola or measles virus).** Rubeola belonging to the **Paramyxoviridae family** is a **nonsegmented, single-stranded, negative sense RNA**

(ss-RNA) virus. The virion is an **enveloped helix.** The ss-RNA is associated with **nucleoprotein (NP),** which maintains the genomic structure, **polymerase phosphoprotein (P protein)**, which facilitates RNA synthesis, and **large protein (L protein)**, which is the **RNA-dependent RNA polymerase.** The viral envelope contains the **fusion protein (F protein)**, which promotes fusion of the envelope to the host cell membrane, **hemagglutinin protein (H protein),** which is a viral attachment protein, and the **matrix protein (M protein),** which is located on the inside of the viral envelope.

3. **Replication**
   a. **Infection and entry.** Rubeola virus infects the host cell through H protein on the viral envelope binding to host cell CD46 protein. The F protein promotes fusion of the viral envelope and the host cell membrane. The nucleocapsid enters the cytoplasm.
   b. **Early transcriptional events.** The viral –RNA is transcribed within the cytoplasm by RNA-dependent RNA polymerase into mRNAs, which are used in the synthesis of six viral proteins (NP, P, L, F, H, M).
   c. **Replication of viral genome.** Viral –RNA replication occurs in the host cell cytoplasm and is mediated by viral RNA-dependent RNA polymerase. The viral –RNA is first transcribed into a +RNA template, which then undergoes replication to form the viral –RNA genome.
   d. **Viral assembly.** The NP, P, and L proteins associate with the viral –RNA genome to form the nucleocapsid. The F and H proteins are inserted into the host cell membrane. The M protein binds to the F and H proteins.
   e. **Viral release.** The nucleocapsid is directed to areas of the host cell membrane, where viral proteins are located. The nucleocapsid associates with the M protein and is released by budding from the host cell membrane.

4. **Identification.** Rubeola can be grown in human and monkey cell cultures. A four-fold increase in antibody titer from the acute to convalescent stage of the disease is diagnostic. Rubeola infections can be identified by histological observation of Giemsa-stained cells from the respiratory tract or urinary sediment that show large, multinucleated giant cells, which contain both an eosinophilic nuclear inclusion body and eosinophilic, irregular cytoplasmic inclusion bodies.

5. **Reservoir.** Rubeola is a highly contagious human pathogen and is transmitted by respiratory droplets before and after the onset of symptoms.

6. **Other diseases. Rubeola or measles** is one of the five classic childhood exanthems, which includes: rubella, roseola, chickenpox, and fifth disease. Measles results from a primary infection with rubeola, whose clinical findings include: fever, cough, coryza (acute rhinitis), conjunctivitis, photophobia, and Koplik's spots (lesions most commonly on the buccal mucosa across the molars). The measles rash starts below the ears, spreads over the body, and is caused by T cells targeted to viral-infected endothelial cells that line small blood vessels.

E. *Mycoplasma pneumoniae*
   1. **General features.** *Mycoplasma pneumoniae* initially causes a **mild upper respiratory tract disease** whose clinical findings include: low-grade fever, malaise, headache, and a hacking cough (initially dry but later productive) that lasts up to 4 weeks. This may then escalate to a **bronchiolitis** showing a neutrophilic exudate within the bronchiolar lumen and a lymphocytic infiltration of the bronchiolar wall. This may then escalate to *Mycoplasma* pneumonia, showing an **interstitial pneumonitis.** *Mycoplasma* pneumonia is referred to as **"walking pneumonia"** and is the **most common pneumonia in school-aged children and young adults.**
   2. **Causative agent (*Mycoplasma pneumoniae*).** The genus *Mycoplasma* are **non-Gram staining bacteria** that are pleomorphic filaments, facultative anaerobic, lack a cell wall (no peptidoglycans), require exogenous sterols to incorporate into their cell membrane, have a generation time of 1–6 hours, form colonies with a fried-egg appearance, and are the smallest, free-living bacteria. *Mycoplasma pneumoniae*

is exceptional in that it is a strict aerobe and forms colonies with a mulberry shape.

3. **Virulence factors.** *Mycoplasma pneumoniae* (an extracellular pathogen) has an adhesion **P1 protein** that allows attachment to the surface of the respiratory epithelium, leading to the destruction of respiratory epithelial cells through the release of hydrogen peroxide, superoxide radicals, and other cytolytic enzymes. *Mycoplasma pneumoniae* functions as a superantigen that stimulates inflammatory cells to the site of infection.

F. *Chlamydia pneumoniae*

1. **General features.** *Chlamydia pneumoniae* causes a mild upper respiratory tract disease whose clinical findings include: persistent cough, malaise, and does not generally require hospitalization. This may then escalate to a pneumonia showing an **interstitial pneumonitis.** *Chlamydia* pneumonia is the **most common pneumonia in adults (18–45 years of age).**

2. **Causative agent (*Chlamydia pneumoniae*).** The genus **Chlamydophila** are **modified Gram-negative bacteria** that have a thin layer of **modified peptidoglycan (no muramic acid)** between their outer and inner membranes, cannot synthesize ATP (i.e., energy parasite), are intracellular pathogens, and have a complex life cycle that includes the **elementary body (EB)** and the **reticulate body (RB).** The **EB** is the infectious, extracellular form that is resistant to drying, metabolically inactive, and binds to epithelial cells through ligands and is phagocytosed. The fusion of endolysosomes with EB-containing phagocytic vacuoles is inhibited so that intracellular killing of the organism does not occur. The **RB** is the intracellular form that is metabolically active, replicates by binary fission, and produces new EBs. Aggregates of RBs (called **inclusion bodies**) can be visualized by fluorescent microscopy.

3. **Identification.** *Chlamydia pneumoniae* is identified by serology when necessary.

4. **Reservoir.** *Chlamydia pneumoniae* is a human pathogen and was first isolated from the conjunctiva of a Taiwanese child. No animal reservoir has been found. *Chlamydia pneumoniae* is transmitted by respiratory droplets. *Chlamydia pneumoniae* has been associated with the pathogenesis of arthrosclerosis.

G. **Psittacosis (parrot fever)**

1. **General features.** *Chlamydia psittaci* causes psittacosis whose clinical findings include: fever, chills, malaise, headache, anorexia, myalgia, arthralgia, pale macular rash, nonproductive cough, rales, and lung consolidation. This may then escalate to a pneumonia showing an **interstitial pneumonitis.** Other systemic clinical findings may include: carditis, hepatomegaly, splenomegaly, and follicular keratoconjunctivitis.

2. **Causative agent (*Chlamydia psittaci*).** The genus **Chlamydophila** is described above (F2).

3. **Identification.** *Chlamydia psittaci* is identified by serology and is not visible with iodine staining.

4. **Reservoir.** *Chlamydia psittaci* is found in virtually all bird species (most commonly parrots, parakeets, cockatiels, and macaws). *Chlamydia psittaci* is transmitted to humans by inhalation of dried bird excrement, urine, or respiratory secretions. Human-to-human transmission is rare.

H. **Q Fever**

1. **General features.** *Coxiella brunetti* causes Q fever whose acute clinical findings include: high fever, chills, severe headache, and myalgia. This may escalate to a pneumonia showing **interstitial pneumonitis** with a mild dry hack or granulomatous hepatitis. There is no rash associated with Q fever. Chronic infection most commonly presents as subacute endocarditis on a prosthetic or previously damaged heat valve. Most cases of Q fever are generally mild, asymptomatic, and self-limiting.

2. **Causative agent (*Coxiella brunetti*).** The genus ***Coxiella*** belonging to the **Rickettsiae family** are **Gram-negative bacilli,** aerobic, and an intracellular pathogen.

3. **Identification.** *Coxiella brunetti* is identified by serology (Weil-Felix is negative). Acute Q fever is diagnosed by high antibody titers against the phase II antigen. Chronic Q fever is diagnosed by high antibody titers against the phase I and phase II antigens. *Coxiella brunetti* is seen best with Giemsa or Gimenez stains.

4. **Reservoir.** *Coxiella brunetti* is found in domestic livestock (particularly sheep, cattle, and goats), reaching high titers in the placenta of infected livestock. Ticks are an important vector in animal transmission but are not a vector in humans. *Coxiella brunetti* is transmitted to humans by inhalation of dust or aerosols of livestock urine, feces, amniotic fluid, or placental tissue.

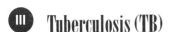 ∅ Ticks

5. **Virulence factors.** *Coxiella brunetti* is highly resistant to desiccation and can remain viable in the environment for months to years. After *Coxiella brunetti* is phagocytosed into the cell, endolysosomes fuse with the *Coxiella brunetti*-containing phagocytic vacuoles and form *Coxiella brunetti*-containing phagolysosomes, but *Coxiella brunetti* survives the acidic environment and is not killed by lysosomal enzymes. *Coxiella brunetti* is able to undergo antigenic modification of the lipopolysaccharide (LPS) endotoxin. The highly infectious form of *Coxiella brunetti* expresses the phase I antigen that blocks antibody interaction with surface proteins. The less infectious form of *Coxiella brunetti* expresses the phase II antigen.[1]

Ⅲ Tuberculosis (TB)

A. Primary TB infection

1. **General features.** *Mycobacterium tuberculosis* causes TB, which is the classic mycobacterial disease. Aerosolized infectious particles travel to terminal airways where *Mycobacterium tuberculosis* penetrates unactivated alveolar macrophages and **inhibits acidification of endolysosomes** so that alveolar macrophages cannot kill the bacteria. However, replicating intracellular *Mycobacterium tuberculosis* stimulates CD8+ cytotoxic T cells, which lyse infected cells and CD4+ helper T cells, which release interferon-γ and other cytokines that activate macrophages to phagocytose and kill the bacteria. The **Ghon complex** is the first lesion of primary TB and consists of a **parenchymal granuloma** (location is **subpleural** and in **lower lobes of the lung**) and **prominent, infected mediastinal lymph nodes.** Most cases of primary TB are asymptomatic and resolve spontaneously.

2. **Causative agent (*Mycobacterium tuberculosis*).** The genus ***Mycobacterium*** are **Gram-positive bacilli** that are poorly Gram-positive bacilli (rods), obligate aerobic, acid-fast (due to a waxy, hydrophobic, arabino-galactan-mycolate cell wall), endospore-negative, nonmotile, and an intracellular pathogen.

3. **Identification.** *Mycobacterium tuberculosis* can be grown in **Lowenstein-Jensen media, Middlebrook media,** and **broths** for rapid, automated testing, the grown colonies have a characteristic **rough, buff appearance,** and the bacterial cells have an **undulating, serpiginous pattern.** *Mycobacterium tuberculosis* **produces niacin, reduces nitrates,** and has a heat-sensitive catalase so that in the standard catalase test (at 68°C), *Mycobacterium tuberculosis* is **catalase-negative.** *Mycobacterium tuberculosis* can be identified by the **purified protein derivative (PPD) skin test** wherein induration is read at 48–72 hours. A positive PPD test only indicates exposure to *Mycobacterium tuberculosis* and cannot by itself distinguish exposure from active disease. *Mycobacterium tuberculosis* can be identified by histological observa-

---

[1]Pneumococcal pneumonia is the most common pneumonia in older adults (>65 years of age).
Viral pneumonia is the most common pneumonia in infants.
Mycoplasma pneumonia is the most common pneumonia in school-aged children and young adults.
Chlamydia pneumonia is the most common pneumonia in adults (18–45 years of age).

tion of the rhodamine–auramine-stained sputum samples demonstrating the stained bacterial cell wall (but is not specific for *Mycobacterium tuberculosis*).

4. **Reservoir.** *Mycobacterium tuberculosis* is found only in humans as the only natural reservoir. *Mycobacterium tuberculosis* is transmitted by aerosolized infectious particles, which travel to terminal airways in the lung.

5. **Virulence factors.** *Mycobacterium tuberculosis* has a cell envelope that contains two factors. **Cord factor (trehalose mycolate)** inhibits mitochondrial respiration and causes virulent *Mycobacterium tuberculosis* to grow in culture as serpentine cords. **Sulfolipids** inhibit acidification of endolysosomes and phagocytic function, which allows *Mycobacterium tuberculosis* to survive intracellularly.

6. **Treatment.** *Mycobacterium tuberculosis* develops drug resistance rapidly when treated with only a single drug. Consequently, treatment of active TB involves the use of multiple drugs. The current standard protocol is: **isoniazid + rifampin + pyrazinamide** for two months, followed by **isoniazid + rifampin** for four more months or until sputum and culture are negative for two consecutive months. If multiple drug-resistant TB is suspected, **ethambutol** or **streptomycin** is added to the above regimen during the first two months.

B. **Secondary (reactivated) TB infection.** During primary TB, large necrotic or caseous granulomas become encapsulated, which effectively seals off the *Mycobacterium tuberculosis* bacteria. The growth of the bacteria is slowed down by the reduced oxygen level, but the bacteria remain viable without prophylactic isoniazid treatment. Later in life if the patient does not receive isoniazid treatment, erosion of a granuloma will release the *Mycobacterium tuberculosis* bacteria into a high oxygen environment and cause secondary or reactivated TB if the person's immune system is reduced as a result of old age or immunosuppressive disease/therapy. This is secondary or reactivated TB and is the most common clinical presentation, usually involving the apical and posterior bronchopulmonary segments of the upper lobes of the lung. Secondary TB spreads via the lymphatics or coughing if cavitation occurs. Clinical findings include: mild fever, night sweats, cough, hemoptysis, weakness, and weight loss.

1. **Cavitary TB.** During secondary TB, diffuse, fibrotic, poorly defined lesions with focal areas of caseous necrosis develop. Often these lesions heal and calcify, but some may erode into a bronchus, creating a tuberculous cavity 3–10 cm in diameter leading to loss of lung parenchyma. The lumen of the cavity is filled with *Mycobacterium tuberculosis* bacteria that may be released into the bronchi and disseminate the infection throughout the lung, especially during coughing.

2. **Miliary TB.** Miliary TB is characterized by numerous, small tuberculous granulomas (1–3 mm in diameter; millet seeds) as a result of dissemination of *Mycobacterium tuberculosis* bacteria throughout the lung (via the lymphatics or airways) or extended to the bone marrow, liver, or spleen (via hematogenous spread).

Ⅳ Thoracic Actinomycosis

A. **General features.** *Actinomyces israeli* causes thoracic actinomycosis, which is characterized by small, multiple, interconnecting lung abscesses. The margins of the abscess are granulomatous while the center is purulent and contains colonies of bacteria called **sulfur granules** which are yellow–orange masses of filamentous bacteria bound together by calcium phosphate.

B. **Causative agent (*Actinomyces israeli*).** The genus ***Actinomyces*** are **Gram-positive bacilli** that are Gram-positive bacilli to branching filamentous forms (similar to hyphae of fungi), anaerobic, non–acid-fast, and endospore-negative.

C. **Identification.** *Actinomyces* can be grown under anaerobic conditions but are slow-growing, fastidious bacteria. The bacterial colonies are white with an irregular, dome-shaped surface that resembles the top of a molar tooth.

D. **Reservoir.** *Actinomyces israeli* normally colonizes mucosal surfaces and is found in gingival crevices and in the female genitourinary (GU) tract. Actinomycosis develops when normal mucosal barriers are disrupted by surgery or trauma so that *Actinomyces israeli* enters normally sterile areas.

E. **Other diseases.** *Actinomyces* is responsible for other diseases, some of which are much more common clinically.
 1. **Cervicofacial actinomycosis.** This is the most common type of actinomycosis and is characterized by facial swelling, fibrosis, scarring, and sinus tracts draining along the angle of the mandible ("lumpy jaw" after tooth extraction).
 2. **Abdominal actinomycosis.** *Actinomyces* may spread throughout the abdomen, potentially infecting every organ.
 3. **Pelvic actinomycosis.** Pelvic actinomycosis is characterized by abscesses of the uterine tube or ovary, ureteral obstruction, or benign vaginitis as a result of using intrauterine devices.
 4. **CNS actinomycosis.** CNS actinomycosis is most commonly characterized by a solitary brain abscess. However, meningitis, subdural empyema, or epidural abscess may also be seen.

V Pulmonary Nocardiosis   Cat +

A. **General features.** *Nocardia asteroides* causes pulmonary nocardiosis, which is characterized by lung abscesses that may show granulomatous features in chronic infections. Pulmonary nocardiosis is frequently seen in patients with lymphomas (low CD4+ helper T cell counts), neutropenia (low leukocyte counts), or HIV infection or in solid organ transplant recipients.

B. **Causative agent (*Nocardia asteroides*).** The genus *Nocardia* are **Gram-positive bacilli** that are poorly Gram-positive bacilli to branching filamentous forms (similar to hyphae of fungi), aerobic, partially acid-fast, catalase-positive, and endospore-negative.

C. **Identification.** *Nocardia* can be grown in most laboratory media but is a slow-growing bacteria (may take a week to isolate). If the specimen for *Nocardia* analysis is potentially contaminated by other bacteria, a buffered charcoal-yeast extract (BCYE) agar may be used. Colonies of *Nocardia asteroides* grown on Middlebrook 7H11 agar show an orange, glabrous, wavy appearance with colonies that tend to adhere to the agar surface. *Nocardia* can be identified by histological observation of bacterially infected tissue or abscess material.

D. **Reservoir.** *Nocardia* is found in soil rich in organic material and is not a component of the normal human flora but rather a transient inhabitant. *Nocardia* is transmitted by inhalation of the bacteria.

VI Fungal Infections

A. Histoplasmosis – silver stains
 1. **General features.** *Histoplasma capsulatum* causes histoplasmosis. Primary histoplasmosis ranges from asymptomatic to an acute, self-limiting fungal pneumonia whose clinical findings include: fever, chills, cough, malaise, headache, myalgia, nausea, and weight loss. This is the most common fungal disease in the United States. Disseminated histoplasmosis occurs in immunocompromised patients as mucocutaneous lesions in the oral and genital areas.
 2. **Causative agent (*Histoplasma capsulatum*).** *Histoplasma capsulatum* is a **thermally dimorphic fungus** with no capsule. The **environmental form** of *Histoplasma capsulatum* is a filamentous (i.e., hyphae) fungus with microspores (microconidia) and

tuberculate macrospores (macroconidia). The tissue form of *Histoplasma capsulatum* is a small 2–4-μm budding yeast cell; relatively uniform in size; has a single bud attached by a narrow base; and found almost exclusively in macrophages.

3. **Identification.** *Histoplasma capsulatum* can be grown in enriched fungal culture media where after 10–30 days of incubation *Histoplasma capsulatum* appears as a silky, hairlike, white–tan mold. *Histoplasma capsulatum* can be identified by the exoantigen test or nuclei acid probe test. A fourfold increase in antibody titer from the acute to convalescent stage of the disease is diagnostic. *Histoplasma capsulatum* infections can be identified by histological observation of Giemsa-stained, Papanicolaou-stained, or methenamine sliver-stained smears and cultures of peripheral blood, bone marrow, and urine.

4. **Reservoir.** *Histoplasma capsulatum* is found in **soil contaminated with bat and bird (starlings and chickens) excreta.** The major endemic areas in the United States are the Ohio, Mississippi, and Missouri rivers beds. *Histoplasma capsulatum* is transmitted by inhalation of spores (conidia) or hyphal fragments during dusty activities where they are phagocytosed by alveolar macrophages, convert to yeasts, and replicate in macrophages.

B. **Coccidioidomycosis (San Joaquin Valley fever)**
   1. **General features.** *Coccidioides immitis* causes coccidioidomycosis. Primary coccidioidomycosis ranges from asymptomatic to an acute, self-limiting fungal pneumonia whose clinical findings include: fever, cough, dull chest pain, and flu-like symptoms. Disseminated coccidioidomycosis occurs in immunocompromised patients, African-Americans and Filipinos, and pregnant women during the third trimester and spreads to the skin, subcutaneous tissues, bones, joints, and meninges.
   2. **Causative agent (*Coccidioides immitis*).** *Coccidioides immitis* is a **thermally dimorphic fungus.** The **environmental form** of *Coccidioides immitis* is a filamentous (i.e., hyphae) fungus that forms arthrospores (arthroconidia) by fragmentation of hyphae. The **tissue form** of *Coccidioides immitis* is a 30–60-μm structure called a spherule that contains 2 to 3 μm endospores.
   3. **Identification.** *Coccidioides immitis* can be grown on conventional media, but cultures are hazardous. *Coccidioides immitis* can be identified by the time-honored tube precipitin test and complement fixation test, although the latex particle agglutination and agar immunodiffusion tests are more sensitive. A fourfold increase in antibody titer from the acute to convalescent stage of the disease is diagnostic. *Coccidioides immitis* can be identified by histological observation of spherules in sputum, urine, or bronchial washings.
   4. **Reservoir.** *Coccidioides immitis* is found in **desert sand.** The major endemic areas in the United States are the San Joaquin Valley in California, Maricopa and Pima counties in Arizona, and southwestern counties of Texas. *Coccidioides immitis* is transmitted by inhalation of arthrospores.

C. **Blastomycosis**
   1. **General features.** *Blastomyces dermatitidis* causes blastomycosis. Primary blastomycosis ranges from asymptomatic to an acute, self-limiting fungal pneumonia and is relatively uncommon. Disseminated blastomycosis spreads to skin and bone.
   2. **Causative agent (*Blastomyces dermatitidis*).** *Blastomyces dermatitidis* is a **thermally dimorphic fungus.** The **environmental form** of *Blastomyces dermatitidis* is a filamentous (i.e., hyphae) fungus with spores (conidia) arising off short, lateral stalks. The **tissue form** of *Blastomyces dermatitidis* is a large 8–15μm yeast cell with a broad base junction between the yeast cells and a thick, double refractive cell wall.
   3. **Identification.** *Blastomyces dermatitidis* can be grown in culture. *Blastomyces dermatitidis* can be identified by histological observation of biopsy specimens demonstrating large yeast cells with a broad base junction between the yeast cells and a thick, double refractive cell wall.

4. **Reservoir.** *Blastomyces dermatitidis* is found in **rotting wood,** although this is uncertain. The major endemic areas in the United States are the Ohio, Mississippi, and Missouri rivers beds (very similar to *Histoplasma capsulatum*), mid-Atlantic region, and northern Minnesota. *Blastomyces dermatitidis* is transmitted by inhalation of spores (conidia).

D. Aspergillosis

1. **General features.** *Aspergillus fumigatus* cause aspergillosis. Invasive aspergillosis is purely an opportunistic infection in immunocompromised patients and is characterized by: patchy focal areas of consolidation, extensive blood vessel invasion leading to infarction of lung tissue, and a fulminant infection not amenable to therapy (rapidly fatal). Aspergilloma is a "fungus ball" that grows in pre-existing lung cavities and is characterized radiographically by a large mass within a lung cavity separated from the wall by air. Allergic bronchopulmonary aspergillosis is an immunological reaction that occurs in asthmatic and allergic persons and is characterized by: transient pulmonary infiltrates, eosinophilia of blood and sputum, increased levels of IgE, and skin sensitivity and serum precipitins to *Aspergillus fumigatus*.

2. **Causative agent (*Aspergillus fumigatus*).** *Aspergillus fumigatus* is a monomorphic, filamentous (i.e., hyphae) fungus with branching hyphae at acute angles [45°] and small 2–4-μm airborne spores (conidia). A specialized hyphal segment forms a conspicuous **fruiting body** from which spores (conidia) are formed.

3. **Identification.** *Aspergillus fumigatus* can be grown on Sabouraud's dextrose agar. *Aspergillus fumigatus* can be identified by histological observation of septate hyphae that branch at regular interval within tissue specimens.

4. **Reservoir.** *Aspergillus fumigatus* is very common in the environment and is found on **almost any moldy organic material** (food, wet ceiling tiles, compost, etc.). *Aspergillus fumigatus* is transmitted by inhalation of spores (conidia).

E. Cryptococcosis   urease ⊕

1. **General features.** *Cryptococcus neoformans* causes cryptococcosis. Primary cryptococcosis ranges from asymptomatic to an acute, self-limiting fungal pneumonia and is characterized by small lung granulomas to several large granulomatous nodules, lung consolidation, and cavitation. Disseminated cryptococcosis is an opportunistic infection in immunocompromised patients, which leads to **cryptococcal meningitis (most common meningitis in AIDS patients),** which is caused by hematogenous spread of the yeast from lung to brain.

2. **Causative agent (*Cryptococcus neoformans*).** *Cryptococcus neoformans* is a monomorphic budding yeast cell with a distinctive acidic polysaccharide capsule that inhibits phagocytosis.

3. **Identification.** *Cryptococcus neoformans* is usually identified in cerebrospinal fluid (CSF) samples. *Cryptococcus neoformans* can be grown on Sabouraud's dextrose agar or niger seed agar and is the only medically important **urease-positive yeast.** *Cryptococcus neoformans* can be identified by the rapid and sensitive latex particle agglutination test, which assays for capsular antigens in the CSF. *Cryptococcus neoformans* can be identified by histological observation of India ink-stained wet mounts of CSF sediments demonstrating budding yeast cells with capsular halos.

4. **Reservoir.** *Cryptococcus neoformans* is found in **soil contaminated with pigeon excreta.** *Cryptococcus neoformans* is transmitted by inhalation of the yeast cells.

F. *Pneumocystis* pneumonia

1. **General features.** *Pneumocystis carinii* causes *Pneumocystis* pneumonia. *Pneumocystis* pneumonia ranges from asymptomatic to an atypical pneumonia showing an **interstitial pneumonitis with plasma cell infiltrates.** Pneumocystis pneumonia is an opportunistic infection in immunocompromised patients (**most common pneumonia in AIDS patients**), premature infants, and malnourished children in close quarters.

2. **Causative agent (*Pneumocystis carinii*).** *Pneumocystis carinii* is obligate extracellular fungus. *Pneumocystis carinii* has various stages in its life cycle: a 1–5-μm trophic form, a 4–5-μm sporocyst, and a 5μm mature spore case that contains 8 spores. When the mature spore case ruptures to release the spores, the spore case wall remains and appears as a collapsed structure or as an empty oval.

3. **Identification.** *Pneumocystis carinii* can be identified by histological observation of Gomori methenamine silver-stained brush biopsy of the lung, needle aspirates of the lung, or bronchoalveolar lavage washings demonstrating the cell wall of 4–5μm sporocysts, which may appear as a dark dot in the center of the sporocyst or as opposing parentheses as a result of local thickenings of the cell wall.

4. **Reservoir.** *Pneumocystis carinii* is very common in the environment, and asymptomatic infections in immunocompetent persons are probably very common whereby the fungus remains dormant for a long time. *Pneumocystis carinii* is transmitted by respiratory droplets and close human contact.

VII Other Respiratory Tract Infections

A. **Croup (Laryngotracheobronchitis)**
1. **General features.** The parainfluenza virus causes croup. Clinical findings include: fever, hoarseness, barking cough and inspiratory stridor, subglottic swelling, airway compression, and respiratory distress. Croup is a common condition in children < 3 years of age. In these children, the larynx is small and the trachea is narrow. When laryngotracheitis occurs, local inflammatory swelling obstructs breathing and causes croup.

2. **Causative agent (parainfluenza virus type 1, 2, 3, 4).** Parainfluenza belonging to the **Paramyxoviridae family** is a **nonsegmented, single-stranded, negative sense RNA (ss-RNA) virus.** The virion is an **enveloped helix.** The ss-RNA is associated with **nucleoprotein (NP),** which maintains the genomic structure, **polymerase phosphoprotein (P protein),** which facilitates RNA synthesis, and **large protein (L protein),** which is the **RNA-dependent RNA polymerase.** The viral envelope contains the **fusion protein (F protein),** which promotes fusion of the envelope to the host cell membrane, **hemagglutinin/neuroaminidase protein (HN protein),** which is a viral attachment protein, and the **matrix protein (M protein),** which is located on the inside of the viral envelope.

3. **Replication**
   a. **Infection and entry.** Parainfluenza virus infects the host cell through HN protein on the viral envelope binding to host cell CD46 protein. The F protein promotes fusion of the viral envelope and the host cell membrane. The nucleocapsid enters the cytoplasm.
   b. **Early transcriptional events.** The viral –RNA is transcribed within the cytoplasm by RNA-dependent RNA polymerase into mRNAs, which are used in the synthesis of six viral proteins (NP, P, L, F, HN, M).
   c. **Replication of viral genome.** Viral –RNA replication occurs in the host cell cytoplasm and is mediated by viral RNA-dependent RNA polymerase. The viral –RNA is first transcribed into a +RNA template, which then undergoes replication to form the viral –RNA genome.
   d. **Viral assembly.** The NP, P, and L proteins associate with the viral –RNA genome to form the nucleocapsid. The F and HN proteins are inserted into the host cell membrane. The M protein binds to the F and HN proteins.
   e. **Viral release.** The nucleocapsid is directed to areas of the host cell membrane where viral proteins are located. The nucleocapsid associates with the M protein and is released by budding from the host cell membrane.

4. **Identification.** Parainfluenza can be grown in primary monkey kidney cells. **Hemadsorption** (adherence of guinea pig RBCs to the parainfluenza virus-infected cultured kidney cells) and **hemagglutination** (aggregation of guinea pig RBCs

when mixed with parainfluenza virus-containing culture media) are nonspecific tests. Specific identification of parainfluenza virus requires **immunological methods** (e.g., immunofluorescence, immunoassays, or specific antibody inhibition of hemadsorption or hemagglutination). Parainfluenza infections can be identified by histological observation of large, multinucleated giant cells. There are four parainfluenza serotypes. Types 1, 2, and 3 are the major causes of croup. Type 4 causes only mild respiratory tract infections in children and adults.

5. **Reservoir.** The parainfluenza virus has a tropism to infect respiratory epithelium. Parainfluenza type 1 and type 2 outbreaks occur mainly in the autumn. Parainfluenza type 3 outbreaks occur throughout the year. The parainfluenza virus spreads readily within hospitals and can cause outbreaks in nurseries and pediatric wards. The parainfluenza virus is transmitted by respiratory droplets and human-to-human contact. Parainfluenza virus is highly contagious and present worldwide.

B. Respiratory syncytial virus (RSV) infection

1. **General features.** Respiratory syncytial virus (RSV) may cause a minor rhinorrhea ("runny nose") in older children and adults or a more severe bronchiolitis in infants and children < 1 year of age. RSV is the most common cause of fatal acute respiratory tract infections in infants and children < 1 year of age. RSV infects nearly every child by 4 years of age. The clinical findings of the more severe bronchiolitis include: low-grade fever, cough, wheezing, tachypnea, tachycardia, air trapping and decreased ventilation as a result of bronchiole inflammation, and respiratory distress.

2. **Causative agent (respiratory syncytial virus; RSV).** RSV belonging to the **Paramyxoviridae family** is a **nonsegmented, single-stranded, negative sense RNA (ss-RNA) virus.** The virion is an **enveloped helix.** The ss-RNA is associated with **nucleoprotein (NP),** which maintains the genomic structure, **polymerase phosphoprotein (P protein),** which facilitates RNA synthesis, and **large protein (L protein),** which is the **RNA-dependent RNA polymerase.** The viral envelope contains the **fusion protein (F protein),** which promotes fusion of the envelope to the host cell membrane, **G protein,** which is a viral attachment protein, and the **matrix protein (M protein),** which is located on the inside of the viral envelope.

3. **Replication**
   a. **Infection and entry.** RSV virus infects the host cell through HN protein on the viral envelope binding to host cell CD46 protein. The F protein promotes fusion of the viral envelope and the host cell membrane. The nucleocapsid enters the cytoplasm.
   b. **Early transcriptional events.** The viral –RNA is transcribed within the cytoplasm by RNA-dependent RNA polymerase into mRNAs, which are used in the synthesis of six viral proteins (NP, P, L, F, G, M).
   c. **Replication of viral genome.** Viral –RNA replication occurs in the host cell cytoplasm and is mediated by viral RNA-dependent RNA polymerase. The viral –RNA is first transcribed into a +RNA template, which then undergoes replication to form the viral –RNA genome.
   d. **Viral assembly.** The NP, P, and L proteins associate with the viral –RNA genome to form the nucleocapsid. The F and G proteins are inserted into the host cell membrane. The M protein binds to the F and G proteins.
   e. **Viral release.** The nucleocapsid is directed to areas of the host cell membrane where viral proteins are located. The nucleocapsid associates with the M protein and is released by budding from the host cell membrane.

4. **Identification.** RSV is difficult to grow in cell culture. RSV can be identified by commercially available immunofluorescent and immunoassay tests of infected cells and nasal washings. RSV infections can be identified by histological observation of large, multinucleated giant cells.

5. **Reservoir.** RSV has a tropism to infect respiratory epithelium. RSV outbreaks occur annually in the winter. RSV spreads readily within nurseries and pediatric wards

with devastating results. RSV is transmitted by respiratory droplets, hands, and human-to-human contact. RSV is highly contagious and present worldwide.

C. Influenza ("the flu")

1. **General features.** Influenza is caused by influenza virus type A and B. Influenza is an acute, highly contagious, self-limiting upper and lower respiratory tract infection. Clinical findings include: rapid onset of fever, chills, myalgia, headache, weakness, and nonproductive cough. The destruction of the ciliated respiratory epithelium may damage the mucociliary elevator and lead to a bacterial pneumonia. The infection may extend down into the lungs causing necrosis of type I pneumocytes and lead to a viral pneumonia (i.e., interstitial pneumonitis).

2. **Causative agent (influenza virus type A and B).** Influenza belonging to the **Orthomyxoviridae virus family** is a **segmented, single-stranded, negative sense RNA (ss-RNA) virus.** The virion is an **enveloped helix** containing eight separate helical segments. The ss-RNA is associated with **nucleoprotein (NP),** which is a component of the nucleocapsid; **nonstructural proteins (NS$_1$ and NS$_2$);** and **RNA-dependent RNA polymerase (PA, PB1, PB2).** The viral envelope contains **hemagglutinin (HA),** which is a viral attachment protein binding to host cell receptors, promotes viral envelope and host cell membrane fusion, agglutinates RBCs, and is the target of neutralizing antibodies; **neuraminidase (NA)** cleaves sialic acid residues of mucus and thereby promotes access to host cells, prevents viral clumping, and facilitates release of virus from infected host cells; **M$_1$ matrix protein** lines the inside of the viral envelope and promotes viral assembly; and **M$_2$ membrane protein** promotes viral uncoating and is a target for the drug amantadine.

3. **Replication**
   a. **Infection and entry.** Influenza virus infects the host cell through HA on the viral envelope binding to host cell membrane receptors, which promotes membrane fusion. The virus enters the host cell cytoplasm by receptor-mediated endocytosis as a coated vesicle and then transferred to an endolysosome. The viral envelope fuses with the endolysosome membrane, and M$_2$ membrane protein promotes viral uncoating, and the nucleocapsid is delivered to the nucleus.
   b. **Early transcriptional events.** The viral −RNA is transcribed within the nucleus by RNA-dependent RNA polymerase into mRNAs, which are used in the synthesis of the viral proteins (NP, NS$_1$, NS$_2$, PA, PB1, PB2, HA, NA, M$_1$, M$_2$).
   c. **Replication of viral genome.** Viral −RNA replication occurs in the host cell nucleus and is mediated by viral RNA-dependent RNA polymerase. The viral −RNA is first transcribed into a +RNA template, which then undergoes replication to form the viral −RNA genome.
   d. **Viral assembly.** The viral −RNA genome is transported to the cytoplasm. The NP, NS$_1$, NS$_2$, PA, PB1, PB2 proteins associate with the viral −RNA genome to form the nucleocapsid. HA and NA are processed by the rER and Golgi and transported by the host cell membrane. M$_1$ and M$_2$ proteins become associated with the host cell membrane.
   e. **Viral release.** The nucleocapsid is directed to areas of the host cell membrane where viral proteins (HA, NA, M$_1$, M$_2$) are located. The virus is released by budding from the host cell membrane.

4. **Identification.** Influenza virus can be grown in primary monkey kidney cells or Madin-Darby canine kidney cells. **Hemadsorption** (adherence of guinea pig RBCs to the influenza virus-infected cultured kidney cells) and **hemagglutination** (aggregation of guinea pig RBCs when mixed with influenza virus-containing culture media) are nonspecific tests. Specific identification of influenza virus requires **immunological methods** (e.g., immunofluorescence, immunoassays, or specific antibody inhibition of hemadsorption or hemagglutination). Influenza type A is classified by type, place of original isolation, date of original isolation, and antigen

(HA, NA) and is designated by the shorthand A/Bangkok/ 1/79 (H3N4). Influenza type B is classified by type, geography, and date of isolation and is designated by the shorthand B/Singapore/ 5/69.

5. **Reservoir.** The influenza virus has a tropism to infect respiratory epithelium. Influenza outbreaks occur annually during winter in people living in temperate climates and are generally present in the community for 4 to 6 weeks. Children, immunosuppressed patients, the elderly, and patients with heart and lung ailments (i.e., smokers) are the most susceptible populations. The influenza virus is transmitted by respiratory droplets expelled during talking, breathing, and coughing. School-age children are most likely to spread the infection.

6. **Virulence Factors**
   a. **Antigenic drift** refers to mutations in the genes for HA or NA viral envelope proteins due to the fact that RNA-dependent RNA polymerase does not have a repair function to correct errors. These mutations produce novel HA and NA viral envelope proteins that result in new strains of influenza virus and cause outbreaks of influenza about every 2 to 3 years. The novel HA and NA viral envelope proteins are designated (H1, H2, H3, etc; N1, N2, N3, etc.). This mandates a vaccine program to protect susceptible individuals from the newest strains of influenza virus.
   b. **Antigenic shift** refers to the reassortment of the eight separate helical segments of ss-RNA between human and animal (e.g., birds, pigs) strains of influenza type A viruses. For example, a pig may be co-infected with a bird influenza type A virus and a human influenza type A virus. In the co-infected pig, reassortment of the eight helical segments of ss-RNA occur such that there are two ss-RNA segments from the bird and six ss-RNA segments from the human. In China, there is close proximity of humans, pigs, ducks, and chickens, which creates a breeding ground for new strains of influenza type A virus that cause pandemics every 10 years or so.

D. **The common cold (coryza)**
   1. **General features.** Rhinovirus and coronavirus cause the common cold. The common cold is an acute, self-limiting upper respiratory tract infection. Clinical findings include: low-grade fever, cough, rhinorrhea, pharyngitis, increased mucus production, nasal congestion, eustachian tube obstruction, and a predisposition to bacterial infections resulting in bacterial sinusitis and otitis media.
   2. **Causative agents (rhinovirus and coronavirus).**
      a. Rhinovirus (at least 100 serotypes) belonging to the **Picornaviridae virus family** is a **nonsegmented, single-stranded, positive sense RNA (ss+RNA) virus.** The virion is a **naked** (nonenveloped) 30-nm **icosahedron.** The Picornaviridae family is divided into two main genera: the **Enterovirus genus** (which includes poliovirus, coxsackievirus, echovirus, enteroviruses 68–71, and hepatitis A, which are acid-stable) and the **Rhinovirus genus** (which consists of at least 100 serotypes of rhinoviruses, which are acid-labile). The rhinovirus has tightly fitting capsomers consisting of four virion proteins (**VP0, VP1-VP4**), which are involved in binding to the host cell. The rhinovirus genome has a 3′ poly A tail that enhances infectivity and a 5′ **VP$_g$ protein** that plays a role in viral RNA packaging into the capsid and initiating viral RNA synthesis. The rhinovirus genome encodes for the capsomers (VP0, VP1-VP4), VP$_g$, at least two proteases, and RNA-dependent RNA polymerase. The rhinovirus is sensitive to acidic pH, is difficult to inactivate with disinfectants or organic solvents, and optimally replicates at **33C,** which limits rhinovirus infection to the cooler upper respiratory tract.
      b. Coronavirus belonging to the **Coronaviridae virus family** is a **nonsegmented, single-stranded, positive sense RNA (ss+RNA) virus.** The virion is an 80–160-nm **enveloped helix,** which resembles a crown (hence the name "corona"). The coronavirus genome encodes for the **E1 protein,** which is a

viral envelope protein, **E2 protein,** which is a viral envelope protein that mediates binding to the host cell, **N protein,** which associates with the viral RNA genome, and a RNA-dependent RNA polymerase. The viral envelope contains prominent surface glycoproteins called hemagglutinins. The coronavirus is sensitive to acidic pH, ether, drying, and optimally replicates at 33C, which limits coronavirus infection to the cooler upper respiratory tract.

3. **Replication**
   a. **Rhinovirus**
      (1) **Infection and entry.** The rhinovirus infects the host cell through **VP1** capsomer protein binding to host cell **ICAM-1** (intercellular adhesion molecule 1). Upon binding VP4 is released and the viral genome is injected directly across the host cell membrane (called **viropexis**).
      (2) **Early transcriptional events.** The viral +RNA is used as mRNA and is translated within the cytoplasm into one large polypeptide, which is cleaved into various viral proteins.
      (3) **Replication of viral genome.** Viral +RNA replication occurs in the host cell cytoplasm and is mediated by RNA-dependent RNA polymerase. The viral +RNA is first transcribed into a –RNA template, which then undergoes replication to the viral +RNA genome. VP_g is attached to the 5′ end.
      (4) **Viral assembly.** The viral proteins (VP0, VP1–VP4) associate to form the capsid and the viral +RNA genome is inserted inside the capsid.
      (5) **Viral release.** The virion is released by cell lysis.
   b. **Coronavirus**
      (1) **Infection and entry.** The coronavirus infects the host cell through E2 viral envelope protein binding to host cell membrane receptors. The nucleocapsid enters the host cell cytoplasm by receptor-mediated endocytosis.
      (2) **Early transcriptional events.** The viral +RNA is used as mRNA and is translated within the cytoplasm into RNA-dependent RNA polymerase. The RNA-dependent RNA polymerase transcribes a –RNA template, which is used for the production of new viral +RNA genome and mRNA. The mRNA codes for various coronavirus proteins.
      (3) **Replication of viral genome.** Viral +RNA replication occurs in the host cell cytoplasm and is mediated by RNA-dependent RNA polymerase. The viral +RNA is first transcribed into a –RNA template, which then undergoes replication to the viral +RNA genome.
      (4) **Viral assembly.** Some viral proteins become associated with the membranes of host cell rough endoplasmic reticulum (rER). Other viral proteins associate with the viral +RNA genome. The viral +RNA genome is enveloped by the viral protein-modified rER and enters the lumen of the rER and travels to the Golgi.
      (5) **Viral release.** Vesicles from the Golgi that contain the enveloped coronavirus migrate to the host cell membrane and are released by budding from the host cell membrane.

4. **Identification**
   a. **Rhinovirus.** The rhinovirus can be grown in human diploid fibroblasts at 33°C. The clinical characteristics of the common cold are so characteristic that laboratory diagnosis is not necessary. Serologic testing to document rhinovirus infection is not practical.
   b. **Coronavirus.** The clinical characteristics of the common cold are so characteristic that laboratory diagnosis is not necessary. Serologic testing to document coronavirus infection is not practical.

5. **Reservoir**
   a. **Rhinovirus.** The rhinovirus has a tropism to infect respiratory epithelium usually in the upper respiratory tract. Rhinovirus cold outbreaks occur most often during early autumn and late spring in people living in temperate climates.

The rhinovirus is transmitted by hands (major vector), respiratory droplets, and human-to-human contact.

b. Coronavirus. The coronavirus has a tropism to infect respiratory epithelium usually in the upper respiratory tract. Coronavirus cold outbreaks occur most often during winter and spring, mainly in infants and children. One strain of coronavirus usually predominates in an outbreak. The coronavirus is transmitted by respiratory droplets.

 Summary Table of Microbiological Diseases Associated With the Lung *(Table 7-1)*

TABLE 7-1	SUMMARY TABLE OF MICROBIOLOGICAL DISEASES ASSOCIATED WITH THE LUNG
Disease	**Microbiological Agent**
Bacterial pneumonia	
Pneumococcal pneumonia	*Streptococcus pneumoniae*
Streptococcal pneumonia	*Streptococcus pyogenes*
Streptococcal pneumonia (newborn)	*Streptococcus agalactiae*
Staphylococcal pneumonia	*Staphylococcus aureus*
Klebsiella pneumonia	*Klebsiella pneumoniae*
Viral and mycoplasma pneumonia	
Cytomegalovirus pneumonia	*Cytomegalovirus*
Varicella pneumonia	*Varicella zoster virus*
Adenovirus pneumonia	*Adenovirus*
Rubeola pneumonia	*Rubeola virus*
Mycoplasma pneumonia	*Mycoplasma pneumoniae*
Chlamydia pneumonia	*Chlamydia pneumoniae*
Psittacosis	*Chlamydia psittaci*
Q fever	*Coxiella brunetti*
Tuberculosis	*Mycobacterium tuberculosis*
Thoracic actinomycosis	*Actinomyces israeli*
Pulmonary nocardiosis	*Nocardia asteroides*
Fungal infections	
Histoplasmosis	*Histoplasma capsulatum*
Coccidioidomycosis	*Coccidioides immitis*
Blastomycosis	*Blastomyces dermatitidis*
Aspergillosis	*Aspergillus fumingatus*
Cryptococcosis	*Cryptococcus neoformans*
Pneumocystis pneumonia	*Pneumocystis carinii*
Other respiratory tract infections	
Croup	*Parainfluenza virus type 1,2,3,4*
Respiratory syncytial virus Infection	*Respiratory syncytial virus*
Influenza	*Influenza virus type A and B*
The common cold	*Rhinovirus* and *Coronavirus*

IX Selected Photographs, Radiographs, and Micrographs

A. **Bacterial pneumonia versus viral pneumonia** (*Fig. 7-1*)

B. **Pneumococcal pneumonia** (*Fig. 7-2*)

C. **Staphylococcal pneumonia** (*Fig. 7-3*)

D. **Viral and mycoplasma pneumonia** (*Fig. 7-4*)

E. **Tuberculosis** (*Fig. 7-5*)

F. **Actinomycosis** (*Fig. 7-6*)

G. **Nocardiosis** (*Fig. 7-7*)

H. **Histoplasmosis** (*Fig. 7-8*)

I. **Coccidioidomycosis** (*Fig. 7-9*)

J. **Blastomycosis** (*Fig. 7-10*)

K. **Aspergillosis** (*Fig. 7-11*)

L. **Cryptococcosis** (*Fig. 7-12*)

M. ***Pneumocystis pneumoniae*** (*Fig. 7-13*)

N. **Mechanisms of Viral Replication** (*Fig. 7-14*)

▶

FIGURE 7-1. **(A) Four stages of bacterial pneumonia. (A-1)** LM of bacterial pneumonia showing macrophages, some neutrophils, fibrin, and edema within the alveoli (*dotted lines*). Bacterial pneumonia is characterized by inflammation within the alveoli. **(B) Four stages of viral pneumonia. (B-1)** LM of viral pneumonia showing mononuclear inflammatory cells (lymphocytes, macrophages, plasma cells), congested capillaries, and edema within the interalveolar septae and pulmonary interstitium (*dotted lines*). Viral pneumonia is characterized by inflammation within the interalveolar septae and pulmonary interstitium. CMV—cytomegalovirus; VZV—varicella-zoster virus.

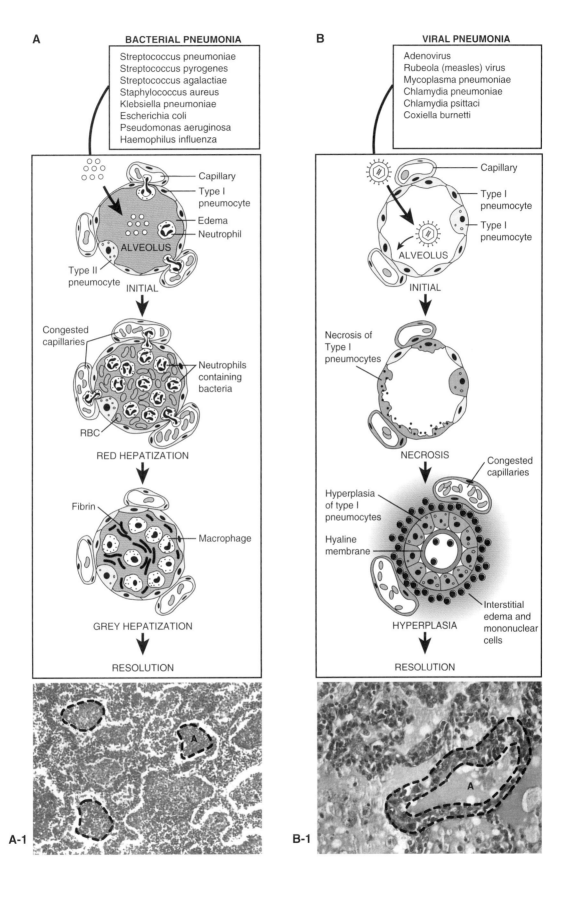

A BACTERIAL PNEUMONIA

Streptococcus pneumoniae
Streptococcus pyrogenes
Streptococcus agalactiae
Staphylococcus aureus
Klebsiella pneumoniae
Escherichia coli
Pseudomonas aeruginosa
Haemophilus influenza

Capillary
Type I pneumocyte
Edema
Neutrophil
ALVEOLUS
Type II pneumocyte
INITIAL

Congested capillaries
Neutrophils containing bacteria
RBC
RED HEPATIZATION

Fibrin
Macrophage
GREY HEPATIZATION

RESOLUTION

A-1

B VIRAL PNEUMONIA

Adenovirus
Rubeola (measles) virus
Mycoplasma pneumoniae
Chlamydia pneumoniae
Chlamydia psittaci
Coxiella burnetti

Capillary
Type I pneumocyte
Type I pneumocyte
ALVEOLUS
INITIAL

Necrosis of Type I pneumocytes
NECROSIS

Congested capillaries
Hyperplasia of type I pneumocytes
Hyaline membrane
Interstitial edema and mononuclear cells
HYPERPLASIA

RESOLUTION

B-1

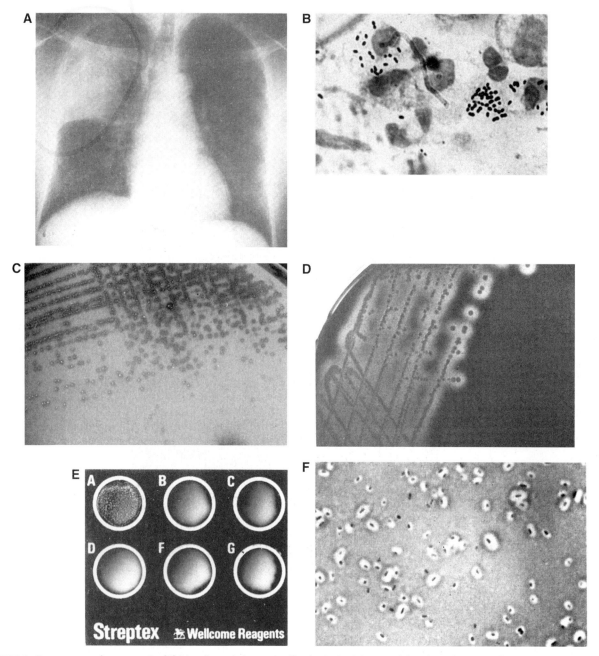

FIGURE 7-2. Pneumococcal pneumonia. (A) PA radiograph shows opacification in the right upper lobe. This radiograph is from a 57-year-old man with fever, chills, and productive cough. Sputum culture was positive for *Streptococcus pneumoniae*. **(B)** LM shows Gram-positive diplococci of *Streptococcus pneumoniae* in a Gram-stained smear of a purulent sputum. Note that neutrophils can also be seen. **(C)** α-hemolytic streptococci (e.g., *Streptococcus pneumoniae*) on sheep blood agar. Streptococci initially may be classified on the basis of their hemolytic properties on sheep blood agar. The partial hemolysis of RBCs results in a greenish zone in the agar medium surrounding the bacterial colonies. **(D)** β-hemolytic streptococci (e.g., *Streptococcus pyogenes*) on sheep blood agar. The complete hemolysis of RBCs results in a clear zone in the agar medium surrounding the bacterial colonies. **(E)** Steptex. The cell wall-grouping antigen is extracted from the bacterial cell wall and incubated with group-specific antibodies bound to latex beads. A positive test is indicated by agglutination of the latex beads as shown in well *A*. Wells *B–G* are negative. **(F)** Quellung reaction. The carbohydrate moieties of the bacterial capsule are incubated with anticapsule antibodies, which cause a refractive change in the capsule such that the capsule appears to "swell."

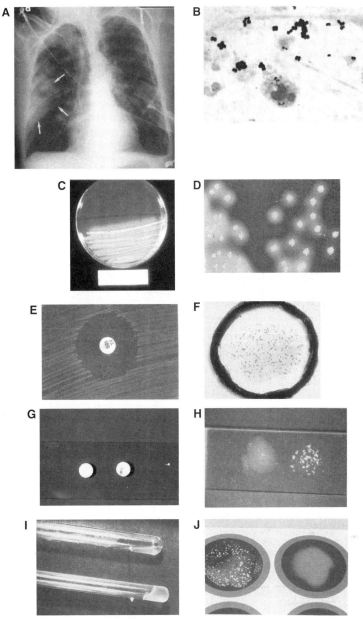

FIGURE 7-3. Staphylococcal pneumonia. (A) *Staphylococcus aureus* septic emboli from an infected central venous catheter. PA radiograph shows a wedge-shaped opacification in the midportion of the right lung (*arrows*) and scattered bilateral nodular opacities. **(B)** LM shows Gram-positive grape-like clusters of *Staphylococci* in a Gram-stained smear of a purulent sputum. Note that a neutrophil can also be seen. **(C)** Mannitol salt agar. Mannitol salt agar is a selective and differential medium used to screen for *Staphylococcus aureus,* which will turn the medium yellow because of its ability to ferment mannitol. **(D)** β-hemolytic *Staphylococcus aureus* on sheep blood agar. The complete hemolysis of RBCs results in a clear zone in the agar medium surrounding the bacterial colonies. **(E)** Furazolidone disk (FX100). The growth of staphylococci is inhibited by furazolidone and shows an area of growth inhibition around the FX 100 disk. **(F)** Passive hemagglutination test. *Staphylococcus aureus* is mixed with sheep RBCs coated with fibrinogen. A positive test is indicated by clumping of the bacteria and RBCs as shown in this figure. **(G)** Modified oxidase test. This is a rapid test to distinguish *Micrococcus* from *Staphylococcus* species. The oxidase reagent is made up in dimethyl sulfoxide to allow penetration into the bacterial cell, and a filter paper disk is rubbed across the bacterial growth. A positive test is indicated by the development of a blue–purple color within 30 seconds. *Micrococcus* species are modified oxidase-positive as indicated by the filter disk on the right. *Staphylococcus* species are modified oxidase-negative as indicated by the filter disk on the left. **(H)** Slide coagulase test. This is a rapid test to identify *Staphylococcus aureus.* The *Staphylococcus aureus* bacteria, which produce a cell-bound coagulase factor, are mixed with EDTA-rabbit plasma. A positive test is indicated by a clumping or agglutination reaction. *Staphylococcus aureus* is coagulase-positive as indicated by the reaction on the right. A negative control is shown on the left. Not all strains of *Staphylococcus aureus* produce a coagulase factor so a negative slide coagulase test must be confirmed by a tube coagulase test. **(I)** Tube coagulase test. The *Staphylococcus aureus* bacteria, which produce an extracellular coagulase factor, are mixed with plasma. The plasma contains a coagulase-reacting factor, which complexes with the coagulase and in turn cleaves fibrinogen to fibrin. A positive test is indicated by the formation of a visible clot. *Staphylococcus aureus* is coagulase-positive as indicated by the reaction in the bottom tube. A negative control is shown in the upper tube. **(J)** Latex agglutination test. The *Staphylococcus aureus* bacteria, which produce coagulase factor and protein A, are mixed with fibrinogen and immunoglobulins bound to latex beads. A positive test is indicated by a clumping or agglutination reaction as indicated in the well on the left. A negative control is shown in the well on the right.

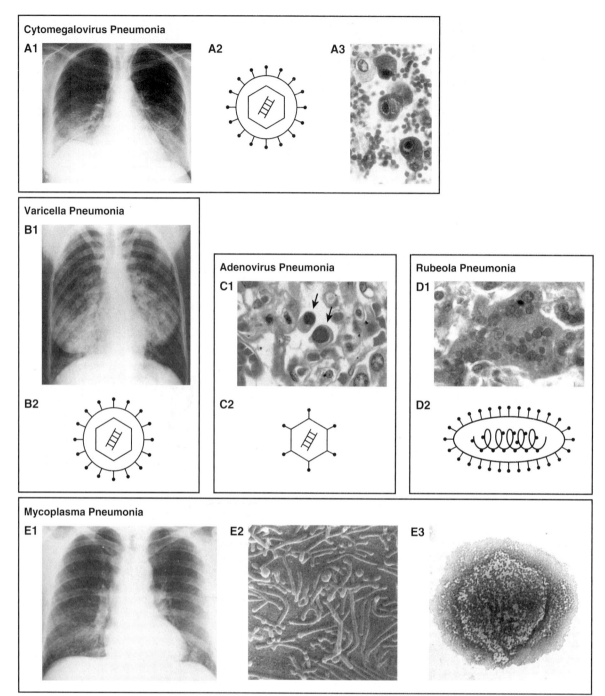

FIGURE 7-4. Viral and mycoplasma pneumonia. (A1, A2, A3) Cytomegalovirus pneumonia. (A1) PA radiograph shows a diffuse reticulonodular pattern involving the midportion and lower portion of both lungs. **(A2)** Diagram of the cytomegalovirus (CMV). CMV is a linear, double-stranded DNA virus that is enveloped and shaped like an icosahedron (approximately 150 nm in diameter). **(A3)** CMV infection is characterized by enlarged cells (i.e., cytomegalic cells), which contain a dense, central, nuclear inclusion body with a peripheral halo (owl's-eye appearance) **(B1 and B2) Varicella pneumonia. (B1)** PA radiograph shows a diffuse acinar nodular pattern with opacification of the perihilar area of both lungs. **(B2)** Diagram of the varicella zoster virus (VZV). VZV is a linear, double-stranded DNA virus that is enveloped and shaped like an icosahedron (about 150 nm in diameter). **(C1 and C2) Adenovirus pneumonia. (C1)** Adenovirus infection is characterized by cells that contain both eosinophilic nuclear inclusion bodies (similar to herpes infections) and indistinct, basophilic nuclear inclusion bodies. These are called smudge cells (*arrows*). **(C2)** Diagram of the adenovirus. Adenoviruses are linear, double-stranded DNA viruses that are naked (nonenveloped) and shaped like icosahedrons (about 70–90 nm in diameter). **(D1 and D2) Rubeola (measles) pneumonia. (D1)** Rubeola infection is characterized by large, multinucleated giant cells, which contain both an eosinophilic nuclear inclusion body and eosinophilic, irregular cytoplasmic inclusion bodies. **(D2)** Diagram of the rubeola or measles virus. The rubeola virus is a nonsegmented, single-stranded, negative sense RNA (ss-RNA) virus that is enveloped and shaped like a helix (about 150–300 nm in diameter). **(E1–E3) Mycoplasma pneumonia. (E1)** PA radiograph shows a diffuse reticulonodular pattern in both lungs. **(E2)** SEM of *Mycoplasma pneumoniae.* Note the pleomorphic filament shaped of the bacteria. **(E3)** A colony of *Mycoplasma pneumoniae.* A single colony of *Mycoplasma pneumoniae* is shown to which sheep RBCs have absorbed to and which generally show a fried-egg appearance. *Mycoplasma pneumoniae* is the only bacteria that demonstrate this RBC-absorbing property.

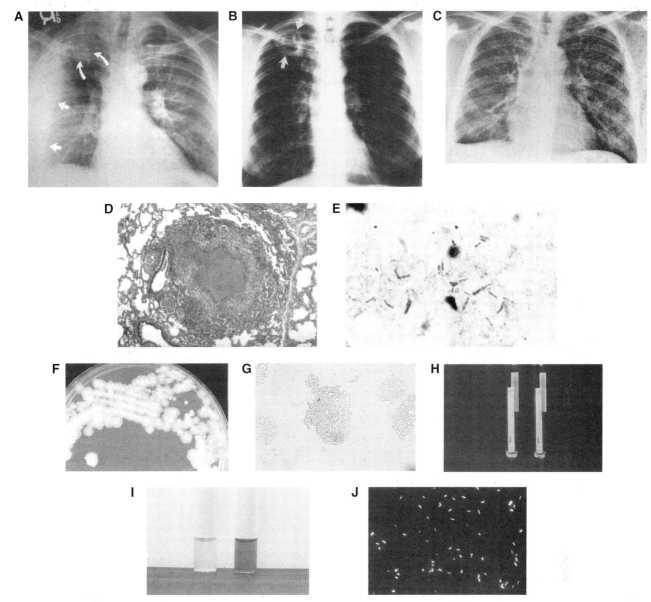

FIGURE 7-5. Tuberculosis. (A) Primary TB. PA radiograph of a 39-year-old man shows an abnormal opacification in the right upper lobe (*curved arrows*) and large right pleural effusion (*straight arrows*) where the pleural fluid collects inferiorly in the upright position and tracks superiorly along the chest wall. **(B)** Cavity TB. PA radiograph shows a cavity in the right upper lobe (*arrows*). **(C)** Miliary TB. PA radiograph shows many small nodules throughout both lungs. **(D)** LM of a small tuberculous granuloma with central caseation found with the lung parenchyma. **(E)** LM shows many red acid-fast bacilli of *Mycobacterium tuberculosis* in an acid-fast stained smear of a purulent sputum. **(F)** Middlebrook 7H10 agar. Colonies of *Mycobacterium tuberculosis* grown on Middlebrook 7H10 agar show a rough, buff appearance. **(G)** LM at low power of a colony of *Mycobacterium tuberculosis* grown on Middlebrook 7H10 agar shows an undulating, serpiginous pattern. **(H)** Niacin accumulation test. The test tubes contain filter paper impregnated with cyanogen bromide and either a fluid extract of *Mycobacterium tuberculosis* or water as a control. A positive test is indicated by the development of a yellow color on the filter paper and in the fluid extract, indicating the presence of niacin. *Mycobacterium tuberculosis* is niacin-positive as indicated by the tube on the right. A negative control is shown on the left. **(I)** Nitrate reduction test. The tube on the right was inoculated with *Mycobacterium tuberculosis* and the tube on the left is the uninoculated control. A positive test is indicated by the development of a red color after the addition of sulfonamide and a-naphthylethylenediamine reagents. *Mycobacterium tuberculosis* is nitrate-positive as indicated by the tube on the right. A negative control is shown on the left. **(J)** LM of a smear from a colony of *Mycobacterium tuberculosis* stained with auramine-rhodamine. Note the brightly stained fluorescence of the short, slightly curved bacilli.

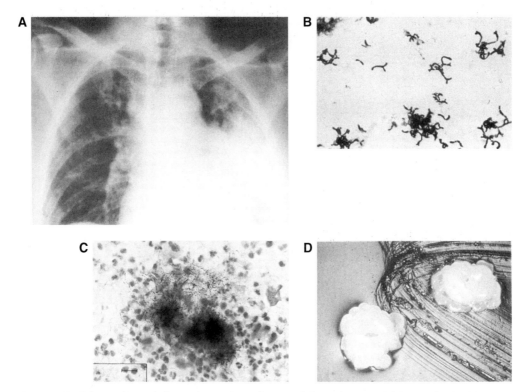

FIGURE 7-6. Actinomycosis. (A) PA radiograph shows abnormal opacification of almost the entire left lung and extending into the chest wall. **(B)** LM shows Gram-positive thin, branching filaments of *Actinomyces israeli.* **(C)** LM shows "sulfur granules," which are yellow–orange masses of filamentous bacteria bound together by calcium phosphate and are characteristic of the *Actinomyces* species. **(D)** Colonies of *Actinomyces israeli* grown on brain–heart infusion agar for seven days at 35°C in anaerobic conditions show a white, irregular, dome-shaped surface that resembles the top of a molar tooth.

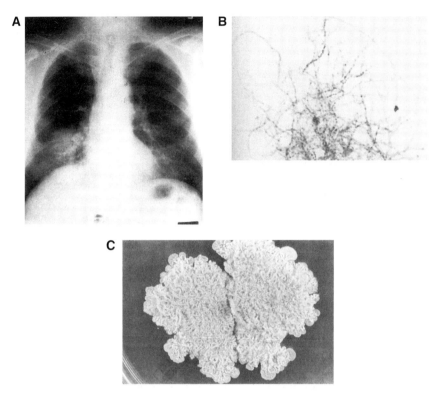

FIGURE 7-7. Nocardiosis. (A) PA radiograph shows a round, dense opacification in the right lower lobe. **(B)** LM (partial acid-fast stain) shows thin, branching filaments of *Nocardia asteroides*. **(C)** Middlebrook 7H11 agar. Colonies of *Nocardia asteroides* grown on Middlebrook 7H11 agar show an orange, glabrous, wavy appearance with colonies that tend to adhere to the agar surface.

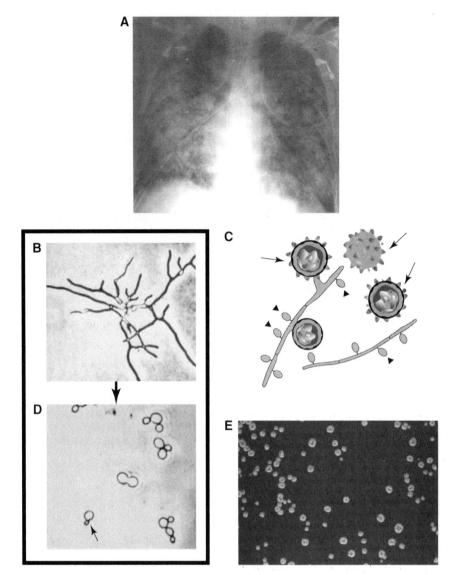

FIGURE 7-8. Histoplasmosis. (A) AP supine radiograph of a 27-year-old man with AIDS shows diffuse, patchy opacification of both lungs. **(B)** LM shows the environmental form of *Histoplasma capsulatum,* which appears as a filamentous (i.e., hyphae) fungus with microconidia (not shown) and macroconidia (not shown). **(C)** Diagram shows the environmental form of *Histoplasma capsulatum,* which appears as a filamentous (i.e., hyphae) fungus with microconidia (*arrowheads*) and macroconidia (*arrows*). **(D)** LM shows the tissue form of *Histoplasma capsulatum,* which appears as small 2–4-μm budding yeast cells that are relatively uniform in size and have a single bud attached by a narrow base (*arrow*). **(E)** 5% sheep blood agar. Colonies of *Histoplasma capsulatum* grown on 5% sheep blood agar show small, yellow yeast cells after conversion from the filamentous fungus form to the yeast cell form. Note that **(B)** and **(D)** show the two different life forms of this thermally dimorphic fungus (in the box).

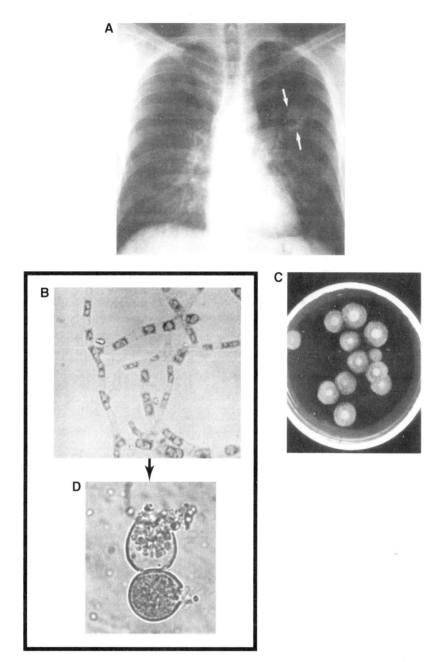

FIGURE 7-9. Coccidioidomycosis. (A) PA radiograph of a 40-year-old man with cough and fever shows a 3-cm cavitary nodule in the upper part of the left lung (*arrows*). **(B)** LM shows the environmental form of *Coccidioides immitis,* which appears as a filamentous (i.e., hyphae) fungus that forms arthrospores (arthroconidia) by fragmentation of hyphae. **(C)** 5% sheep blood agar. Colonies of *Coccidioides immitis* grown on 5% sheep blood agar show gray–white, delicate hair-like appearance. This is the environmental form of *Coccidioides immitis.* **(D)** LM shows the tissue form of *Coccidioides immitis,* which appears as a 30–60-µm spherule that contains 2–3-µm endospores. Note the two spherules that have ruptured to release the endospores. Note that **(B)** and **(D)** show the two different life forms of this thermally dimorphic fungus (in the box).

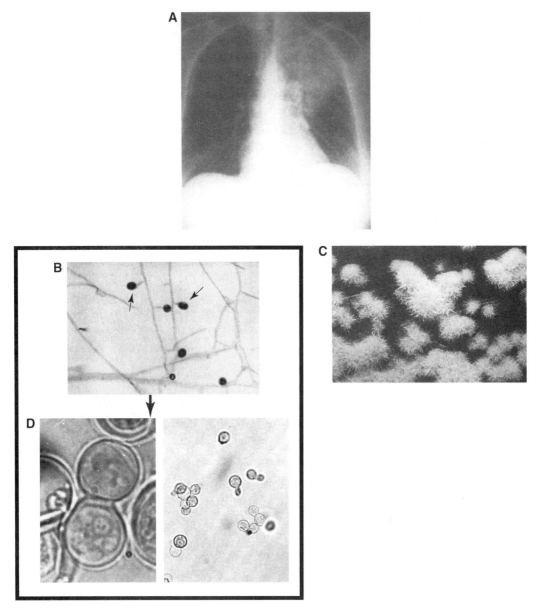

FIGURE 7-10. Blastomycosis. (A) PA radiograph of a 53-year-old woman with a productive cough shows an opacification in the left upper lobe. **(B)** LM shows the environmental form of *Blastomyces dermatitidis,* which appears as a filamentous (i.e., hyphae) fungus with spores (conidia; *arrows*) arising off short, lateral stalks resembling a lollipop appearance. **(C)** 5% sheep blood agar. Colonies of *Blastomyces dermatitidis immitis* grown on 5% sheep blood agar at 37°C show a white, coarse spicule appearance. This is called the "prickly form," which is an intermediate stage between the environmental form and tissue form. **(D)** LM shows the tissue form of *Blastomyces dermatitidis,* which appears as a large 8–15-μm yeast cell with a broad base junction between the yeast cells and a thick, double refractive cell wall. Both high and low magnifications are shown. Note that **(B)** and **(D)** show the two different life forms of this thermally dimorphic fungus (in the box).

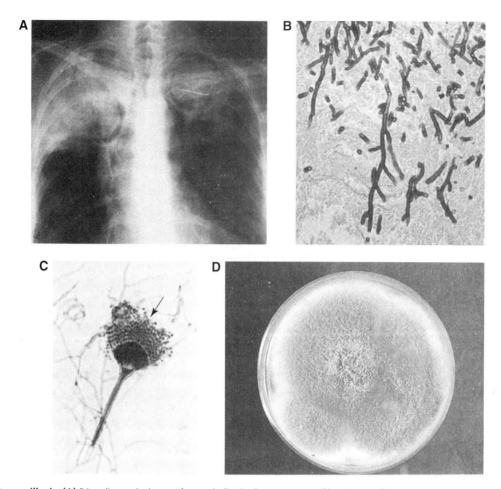

FIGURE 7-11. Aspergillosis. (A) PA radiograph shows "fungus balls" in the upper part of both lungs. **(B)** LM shows *Aspergillus fumingatus,* which appears as a monomorphic, filamentous (i.e., hyphae) fungus with branching hyphae at acute angles. **(C)** LM shows the fruiting body of *Aspergillus fumingatus.* A specialized hyphal segment called the *foot cell* serves as the origin of the conidiophore. The formation of spores (conidia) occurs in the fruiting body. The fruiting body consists of a swollen vesicle and one or two rows of phialides, which give rise to rows of pigmented spores (conidia; *arrows*). **(D)** Sabouraud's dextrose agar. Colonies of *Aspergillus fumingatus* grown on Sabouraud's dextrose agar show a green, powdery appearance. The growing margin of the fungus appears as a "white apron."

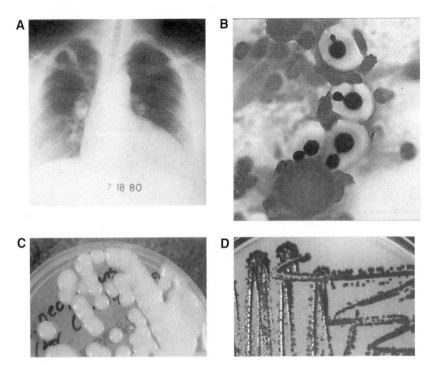

FIGURE 7-12. Cryptococcosis. (A) PA radiograph of a transplant recipient shows opacifications in both lungs. **(B)** LM shows *Cryptococcus neoformans* from a bronchoalveolar lavage, which appears as a budding yeast cell (*arrow;* black) surrounded by a thick polysaccharide capsule (*arrowhead;* clear area). **(C)** Sabouraud's dextrose agar. Colonies of *Cryptococcus neoformans* grown on Sabouraud's dextrose agar show a white, mucoid appearance. **(D)** Niger see agar. Colonies of *Cryptococcus neoformans* grown on niger seed agar show maroon–red appearance.

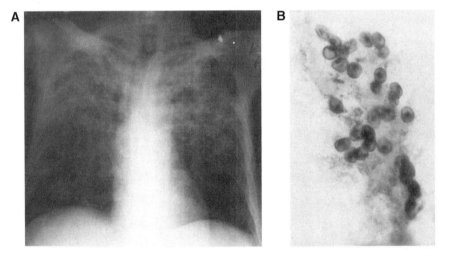

FIGURE 7-13. Pneumocystis pneumoniae. (A) PA radiograph of a 41-year-old man with AIDS shows interstitial and alveolar opacification in the upper part of both lungs. **(B)** LM shows *Pneumocystis carinii* from a Gomori methenamine silver-stained bronchoalveolar lavage, which appears as 4–5-μm sporocysts. The Gomori methenamine silver-stain impregnates the cell wall, which appears either as a dark dot in the center of the sporocyst or as opposing parentheses as a result of local thickenings of the cell wall. Note that the dark dot is not the nucleus of the sporocyst.

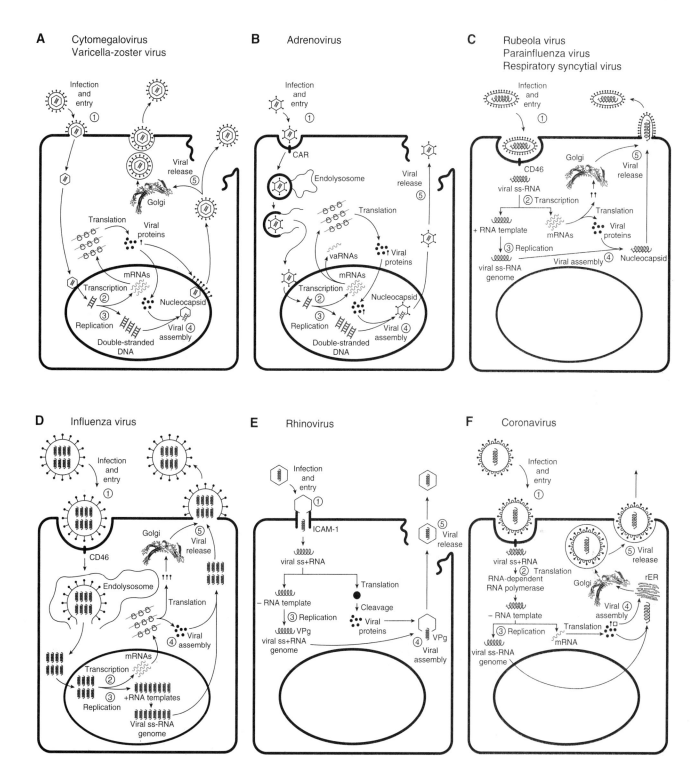

FIGURE 7-14. Mechanisms of viral replication. (A) Cytomegalovirus (CMV) and varicella zoster virus (VZV). These viruses are enveloped, linear, double-stranded DNA viruses. See IIA3 and IIB3 for explanation. **(B)** Adenovirus. This virus is a naked, linear, double-stranded DNA virus. See IIC3 for explanation. **(C)** Rubeola virus, parainfluenza virus, and respiratory syncytial virus (RSV). These viruses are enveloped, nonsegmented, single-stranded negative-sense RNA viruses. See IID3, VIIA3, and VIIB3 for explanations. **(D)** Influenza virus. This virus is an enveloped, segmented, single-stranded negative sense RNA virus. See VIIC3 for explanation. **(E)** Rhinovirus. This virus is a naked, nonsegmented, single-stranded positive-sense RNA virus. See VIID3a for explanation. **(F)** Coronavirus. This virus is an enveloped, nonsegmented, single-stranded positive-sense RNA virus. See VIID3b for explanation. CAR—Coxsackie adenovirus receptor; ICAM-1—intercellular adhesion molecule-1; vaRNA—virus-associated RNA segments; ss-RNA—single-stranded negative-sense RNA.

Chapter 8

Pharmacology

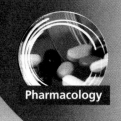

Pharmacology

I Antiasthmatic Drugs (Fig. 8-1)

A. **Terbutaline, albuterol, metaproterenol,** and **salmeterol** are β_2-**adrenergic** receptor agonists (i.e., β_2-**agonists**) that promote bronchodilation (i.e., relaxation of bronchial smooth muscle). In asthma, the FEV_1 (the volume of air that can be expired in one second following a maximal inspiration) is reduced. After treatment with a β_2-agonist, the FEV_1 is increased. The β_2-adrenergic receptor is a **G-protein linked receptor** that works through the **adenylate cyclase pathway** as follows: when epinephrine (E) binds to the β_2 receptor, **inactive G_S** protein (which exists as a trimer with GDP bound to the α_S chain) exchanges its GDP for GTP to become **active G_S** protein. This allows the α_S chain to disassociate from the β_S chain and γ_S chain and **stimulate adenylate cyclase to increase cAMP levels.** Active G_S protein is short-lived since the α_S chain has **GTPase activity,** which quickly hydrolyzes GTP to GDP to form inactive G_S protein.

cAMP activates the enzyme **cAMP-dependent protein kinase (or protein kinase A; PKA),** which catalyzes the **covalent phosphorylation** of serine and threonine within certain intracellular proteins to increase their activity. This results in the following cellular responses: **a decrease in intracellular Ca^{2+}, inactivation of myosin kinase, and opening of maxi-K^+ channels (membrane large conductance calcium-activated potassium channels).** The enzyme **serine/threonine protein phosphatase** reverses the effects of protein kinase A by dephosphorylation of serine and threonine.

B. **Atropine and ipratropium** are **M_3 muscarinic acetylcholine receptor (M_3AChR) antagonists that inhibit bronchoconstriction** (i.e., contraction of bronchial smooth muscle). The M_3AChR is a G-protein linked receptor that works through the **phospholipase C pathway** as follows: when acetylcholine (Ach) binds to M_3AChR, **inactive G_q** protein (which exists as a trimer with GDP bound to the α chain) exchanges its GDP for GTP to become **active G_q protein.** Active G_q protein activates **phospholipase C,** which cleaves **phosphatidylinositol biphosphate (PIP_2)** into **inositol triphosphate (IP_3)** and **diacylglycerol (DAG).**

IP_3 causes the **release of Ca^{++} from the smooth endoplasmic reticulum,** which activates the enzyme **Ca^{++}/calmodulin-dependent protein kinase (or CaM-kinase),** which catalyzes the **covalent phosphorylation** of serine and threonine within certain intracellular proteins to increase their activity. DAG activates the enzyme **protein kinase C (PKC),** which catalyzes the **covalent phosphorylation** of serine and threonine within certain intracellular proteins to increase their activity. This results in the following cellular responses: **an increase in intracellular Ca^{2+}, activation of myosin kinase, and closure of maxi-K^+ channels (membrane large conductance calcium-activated potassium channels).** The enzyme **serine/threonine protein phosphatase** reverses the effects of CaM-kinase and PKC A by dephosphorylation of serine and threonine.

C. **Cromolyn (NasalCrom)** inhibits the release of histamine from mast cells.

D. **Beclomethasone, budesonide,** and **triamcinolone** are corticosteroids that have an anti-inflammatory effect by reducing the synthesis of arachidonic acid by phospholipase A_2 and inhibiting the expression of cyclooxygenase II (COX II).

119

A

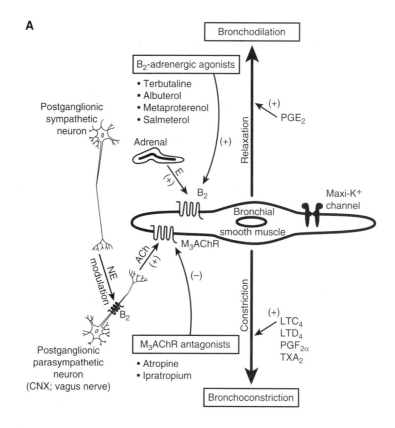

B

C

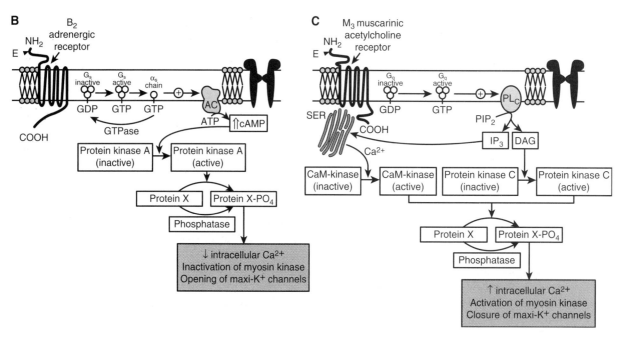

FIGURE 8-1. (A) Diagram indicating the various factors that control bronchial smooth muscle relaxation and contraction. Note that epinephrine from the adrenal medulla, PGE_2, and β_2-adrenergic agonists (e.g., terbutaline, albuterol, metaproterenol, salmeterol) promote bronchodilation. Note that postganglionic parasympathetic neurons through the release of acetylcholine (ACh), leukotrienes (LTC_4, LTD_4), $PGF_{2\alpha}$, and thromboxane (TXA_2) promote bronchoconstriction. The M_3AChR antagonists (e.g., atropine and ipratropium) block the bronchoconstrictive action of ACh. Note that postganglionic sympathetic neurons do not affect bronchial smooth muscle directly. Instead, postganglionic sympathetic neurons terminate on postganglionic parasympathetic neurons and modulate their bronchoconstrictive action (see Gross Anatomy IIIF). **(B) Diagram of the β_2-adrenergic receptor action that works through the adenylate cyclase pathway.** See text for explanation. **(C) Diagram of the M_3 muscarinic acetylcholine receptor action that works through the phospholipase C pathway.** See text for explanation. a_s—alpha chain; AC—adenylate cyclase; ATP—adenosine triphosphate; cAMP—cyclic adenosine monophosphate; E—epinephrine; DAG—diacylglycerol; GDP—guanosine diphosphate; G_q—protein that stimulates phospholipase C; G_s—protein that simulates adenylate cyclase; GTP—guanosine triphosphate; M_3AChR—M_3 muscarinic acetylcholine receptor; NE—norepinephrine; PIP 2—phosphatidylinositol biphosphate; SER—smooth endoplasmic reticulum.

Allergies, Seasonal Hay Fever, Rhinitis, and Urticaria

Allergies, seasonal hay fever, rhinitis, and urticaria can be treated with the following drugs:

A. Diphenhydramine (Benadryl), dimenhydrinate (Dramamine), chlorpheniramine (Chlor-Trimeton), and meclizine (Antivert) are first-generation H_1-receptor antagonists that block the effect of histamine released from mast cells on vascular permeability, vasodilation, and smooth muscle contraction of bronchi. The H_1-receptor is a G-protein linked receptor that increases IP_3 and DAG levels.

B. Fexofenadine (Allegra), desloratadine (Clarinex), and cetirizine (Zyrtec) are second-generation H_1-receptor antagonists. These drugs do not cross the blood–brain barrier and therefore do not have a sedative effect like the first-generation drugs listed above.

III Antibiotics (Fig. 8-2)

Antibiotics are chemical substances produced by certain microorganisms (e.g., bacteria, fungi, actinomycetes) that either arrest the growth and replication of bacteria (i.e., bacteriostatic) or kill the bacteria (i.e., bacteriocidal). Antibiotics can be classified according to their actions, which include: cell wall inhibitors and β-lactamase inhibitors; protein synthesis inhibitors; DNA replication inhibitors; and metabolic inhibitors.

A. Cell wall synthesis inhibitors

1. **Natural penicillins [penicillin G (Pfizerpen), penicillin V (V-Cillin K), penicillin G procaine (Duracillin A.S.), penicillin G benzathine (Bicillin L-A)].** Penicillin is a bacteriocidal agent whose active nucleus is a four-membered ring called the β-**lactam ring. The mechanism of action is:** attachment to specific penicillin-binding proteins located on the bacterial cell membrane and inhibition of transpeptidation or carboxypeptidation of peptidoglycan moieties of the bacterial cell wall. This reduces the cross-linking of the cell wall and the bacteria rupture as a result of the high internal osmotic pressure. **The mechanism of resistance is:** production by the bacteria of penicillinase or β-lactamase enzymes that split the β-lactam ring of penicillin. **Clinical uses include:** Gram-positive, Gram-negative, spirochetes, and anaerobic coverage; pneumonia caused by *Streptococcus pneumoniae*; gingivostomatitis caused by *Leptotrichia buccalis*; syphilis caused by *Treponema pallidum*; actinomycosis caused by *Actinomyces israelii*; diphtheria caused by *Corynebacterium diphtheria*; anthrax caused by *Bacillus anthracis*; gas gangrene caused by *Clostridium perfringens*; *Streptococcus pyogenes* infections; and *Neisseria meningitis* infections.

2. **Antistaphylococcal penicillins [methicillin (Staphcillin), nafcillin (Unipen), oxacillin (Bactocill), dicloxacillin (Dynapen), cloxacillin (Tegopen)]** are penicillinase-resistant. **Clinical uses include:** a narrow spectrum of use against penicillinase-producing *Staphylococci* and ineffective against Gram-negative bacteria.

3. **Aminopenicillins [ampicillin (Omnipen), amoxicillin (Amoxil)]** are inactivated by β-lactamases and are therefore often combined with β-lactamase inhibitors clavulanic acid (Augmentin) or sulbactam (Unasyn). **Clinical uses include:** Gram-negative bacteria coverage; upper respiratory tract infections caused by *Streptococcus pneumoniae, Streptococcus pyogenes,* and *Haemophilus influenzae*; urinary tract infections caused by Group D enterococci; bacterial meningitis caused by *Listeria monocytogenes*; and invasive *Salmonella* infections.

4. **Antipseudomonal penicillins [mezlocillin (Mezlin), piperacillin (Pipracil), azlocillin (Azlin), carbenicillin (Geopen), ticarcillin (Ticar)]** are destroyed by β-lactamases. **Clinical uses include:** Gram-negative bacilli coverage and serious *Pseudomonas* infections.

5. **First-generation cephalosporins [cephalothin (Keflin), cephapirin (Cefadyl), cephradine (Velosef), cephalexin (Keflex), cefazolin (Ancef), cefadroxil**

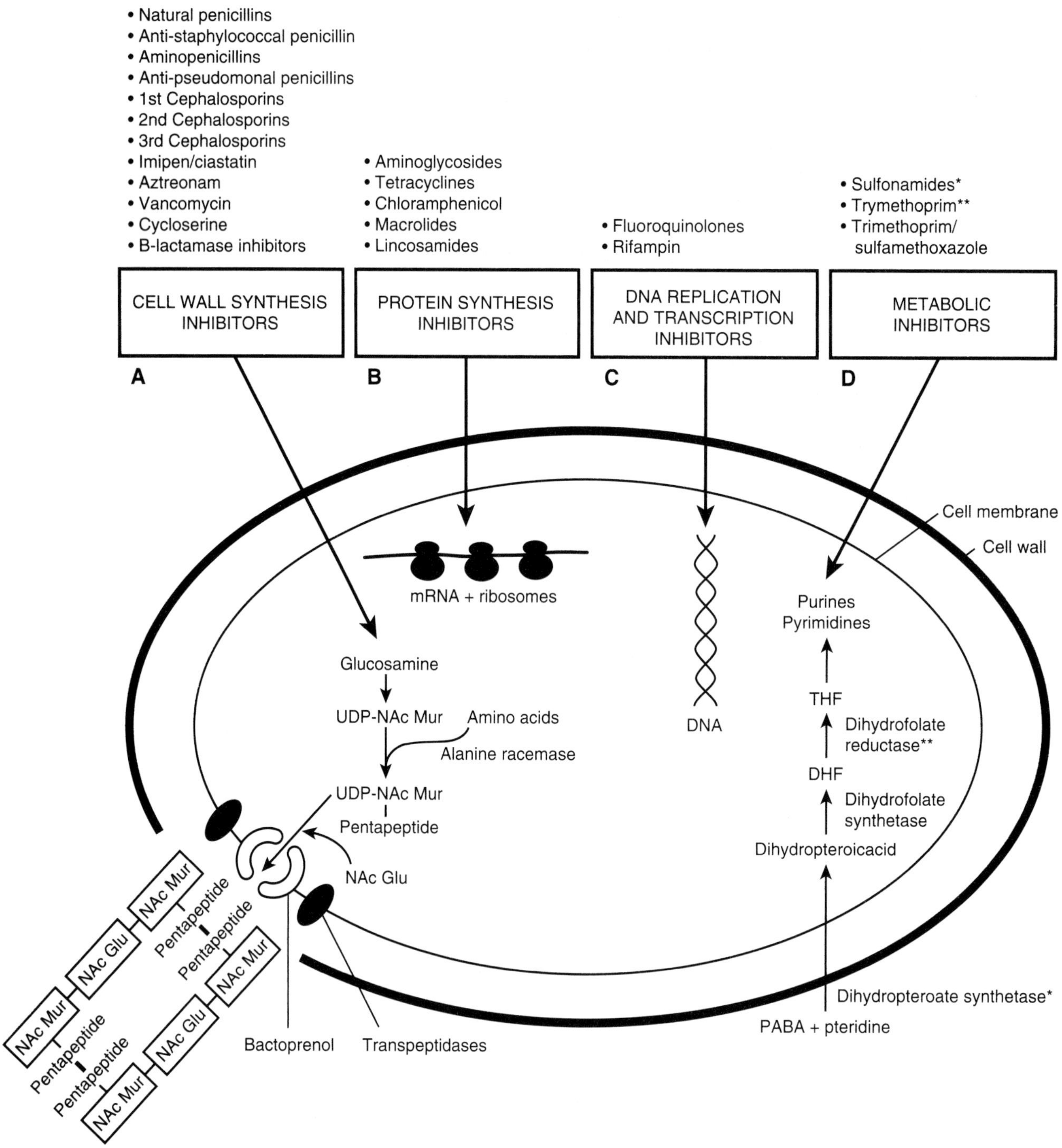

- Natural penicillins
- Anti-staphylococcal penicillin
- Aminopenicillins
- Anti-pseudomonal penicillins
- 1st Cephalosporins
- 2nd Cephalosporins
- 3rd Cephalosporins
- Imipen/ciastatin
- Aztreonam
- Vancomycin
- Cycloserine
- B-lactamase inhibitors

- Aminoglycosides
- Tetracyclines
- Chloramphenicol
- Macrolides
- Lincosamides

- Fluoroquinolones
- Rifampin

- Sulfonamides*
- Trymethoprim**
- Trimethoprim/
  sulfamethoxazole

CELL WALL SYNTHESIS INHIBITORS	PROTEIN SYNTHESIS INHIBITORS	DNA REPLICATION AND TRANSCRIPTION INHIBITORS	METABOLIC INHIBITORS
A	B	C	D

Cell membrane
Cell wall

mRNA + ribosomes

Glucosamine

UDP-NAc Mur   Amino acids

Alanine racemase

UDP-NAc Mur
|
Pentapeptide

NAc Glu

DNA

Purines
Pyrimidines

THF

Dihydrofolate
reductase**

DHF

Dihydrofolate
synthetase

Dihydropteroicacid

NAc Mur

NAc Glu

Pentapeptide

Bactoprenol   Transpeptidases

Dihydropteroate synthetase*

PABA + pteridine

FIGURE 8-2. Pharmacological site of action of antibiotics. (A) Cell wall synthesis inhibitors. The synthesis of the bacterial cell wall is a complicated process involving peptidoglycan, which is a mesh of polysaccharide chains cross-linked by peptides. The polysaccharides are repeating units of N-acetylglucosamine (NAcGlu) and N-acetylmuramic acid (NAcMur). There are four basic steps in peptidoglycan synthesis: 1. Glucosamine is converted to NAcMur and then activated by uridine triphosphate (UTP) to produce UDP-NAcMur. A pentapeptide is attached to UDP-NAcMur by alanine racemase to form UDP-NAcMur-pentapeptide. 2. UDP-NAcMur-pentapeptide is attached to bactoprenol (a carrier protein) and NAcGlu is added to form NAcGlu–UDP-NAcMur-pentapeptide. 3. NAcGlu–UDP-NAcMur-pentapeptide is transported out of the bacteria by bactoprenol and is linked to other peptidoglycans in the cell wall. 4. The pentapeptide chains are cross-linked by transpeptidases, which determines the strength and rigidity of the cell wall. **(B) Protein synthesis inhibitors. (C) DNA replication and transcription inhibitors. (D) Metabolic inhibitors.** The pathway of folic acid synthesis involves a number of reactions leading to the production of purines and pyrimidines. DHF—dihydrofolate; THF—tetrahydrofolate; *—site of action for sulfonamides; **—site of action for trimethoprim.

(Duricef)]. The structure of cephalosporins is very similar to the structure of penicillins, both of which have a β-lactam ring and a dihydrothiazine ring. The mechanism of action is similar to the penicillins. However, the cephalosporins have a broader antibacterial spectrum and are more resistant to β-lactamases than are the penicillins. The first-generation cephalosporins penetrate most tissues effectively but do not penetrate the central nervous system (CNS) and therefore are not used to treat meningitis. **Clinical uses include:** Gram-positive coverage excellent, Gram-negative and anaerobic coverage poor; pneumonia caused by *Klebsiella pneumoniae*; endocarditis caused by *Staphylococcus aureus*; urinary tract infections caused by *Escherichia coli*, *Proteus*, and *Klebsiella*; surgical prophylaxis; *Streptococci* infections; Proteus mirabilis infections; and *Peptococcus* and *Peptostreptococcus* infections.

6. **Second-generation cephalosporins [cefamandole (Mandol), cefaclor (Ceclor), cefoxitin (Mefoxin), cefotetan (Cefotan), cefonicid (Monocid), cefprozil (Cefzil), cefuroxime (Ceftin), cefpodoxime proxetil (Vantin)].** In comparison with first-generation cephalosporins, second-generation cephalosporins have a broader spectrum, are more resistant to β-lactamases, and have a limited penetration of the CNS. **Clinical uses include:** Gram-positive coverage decreased, Gram-negative coverage increased, and anaerobic coverage moderate; sepsis or peritonitis caused by *Bacteroides fragilis* (drugs of choice: cefotetan and cefoxitin); meningitis caused by *Haemophilus influenzae*, *Neisseria meningitidis*, and *Streptococcus pneumoniae* (drug of choice: cefuroxime); pneumoniae caused by *Klebsiella pneumonia*; urinary tract infections; sinusitis; otitis media; bone and soft tissue infections; *Enterobacter aerogenes*, *Proteus mirabilis*, *Escherichia coli*, and *Serratia* infections.

7. **Third-generation cephalosporins [ceftriaxone (Rocephin), ceftazidime (Fortaz), cefotaxime (Claforan), ceftizoxime (Cefizox), moxalactam (Moxam), cefixime (Suprax), cefoperazone (Cefobid)].** In comparison with first- and second-generation cephalosporins, third-generation cephalosporins have the broadest spectrum, are the most resistant to β-lactamases, have the best penetration of the CNS, and have the highest lipid solubility. **Clinical uses include:** Gram-positive coverage poor, Gram-negative coverage excellent, anaerobic coverage moderate; meningitis caused by *Haemophilus influenzae*, *Neisseria meningitidis*, and *Streptococcus pneumoniae* (drug of choice: ceftriaxone); pneumonia and sinusitis caused by *Streptococcus pneumoniae*; gonorrhea caused by *Neisseria gonorrhoeae* (drug of choice: ceftriaxone); Lyme disease (2nd stage) caused by *Borrelia burgdorferi* (drug of choice: ceftriaxone); chancroid caused by *Haemophilus ducreyi*; urinary tract infections caused by *Pseudomonas aeruginosa*, *Proteus*, and *Klebsiella*; and *Salmonella*, *Serratia*, *Enterobacter*, and *Bacteroides fragilis* infections.

8. **Imipenem/cilastatin (Primaxin).** Imipenem is carbapenem derived from *Streptococcus cattleya* whose mechanism of action is similar to the penicillins and cephalosporins. Imipenem is resistant to most β-lactamases and penetrates most tissues, including the CNS. Imipenem is metabolized in the kidney by dehydropeptidases that produce a nephrotoxic metabolite. Imipenem is always administered with cilastatin, which inhibits the dehydropeptidases and eliminates the nephrotoxicity. **Clinical uses include:** Gram-positive and Gram-negative coverage both aerobic and anaerobic; broadest spectrum β-lactam antibiotic currently available.

9. **Aztreonam (Azactam).** Aztreonam is a monobactam derived from *Chromobacterium violaceum* whose mechanism of action is similar to the penicillins and cephalosporins. Aztreonam is extremely resistant to most β-lactamases. **Clinical uses include:** no Gram-positive coverage, Gram-negative aerobic bacilli coverage excellent, no anaerobic coverage; *Enterobacter*, *Pseudomonas aeruginosa*, and *Serratia* infections.

10. **Vancomycin (Vancocin).** Vancomycin is tricyclic glycopeptide derived from *Streptomyces orientalis*. **The mechanism of action is:** binding to D-alanyl D-alanine terminus of the pentapeptide in Gram-positive bacterial cell wall precursors

that prevents transpeptidation (this mechanism of action is at a step earlier than the mechanism of action of penicillin). **The mechanism of resistance is:** plasmid-mediated and decreased binding to receptor molecules. **Clinical uses include:** Gram-positive coverage excellent, especially against methicillin-resistant *Staphylococcus aureus* (MRSA), multidrug-resistant *Staphylococcus epidermidis* (MRSE), and *Enterococcus faecalis* (group D streptococcus); no Gram-negative coverage; pseudomembranous colitis caused by *Clostridium difficile;* and prophylaxis in patients with prosthetic heart valves undergoing dental procedures.

11. **Cycloserine (Seromycin).** Cycloserine is a structural analogue of alanine derived from *Streptococcus orchidaceus.* **The mechanism of action is:** as an analogue of alanine, cycloserine inhibits **alanine racemase,** which prevents bacterial cell wall synthesis. Cycloserine penetrates most tissues and fluids effectively, including the CNS. **Clinical uses include:** Gram-positive coverage good, Gram-negative coverage good, but used primarily against *Mycobacterium;* tuberculosis caused by *Mycobacterium tuberculosis* used in combination with other drugs.

12. **β-lactamase inhibitors [clavulanic acid (Augmentin), sulbactam (Unasyn), tazobactam].** **The mechanism of action is:** irreversible binding to and inactivation of β-lactamases, thereby preventing them from destroying β-lactam antibiotics. **Clinical uses include:** to prevent hydrolyzable penicillins from destruction by β-lactamases.

13. **Cefepime (Maxipime). The mechanism of action is:** attachment to specific penicillin-binding proteins located on the bacterial cell membrane and inhibition of transpeptidation or carboxypeptidation of peptidoglycan moieties of the bacterial cell wall. **Clinical uses include:** wide coverage of Gram-positive and Gram-negative bacteria.

B. Protein synthesis inhibitors

1. **Aminoglycosides.** Aminoglycosides are amino sugars linked to an aminocyclitol ring by glycosidic bonds derived from various species of *Streptomyces.* **The mechanism of action is:** aminoglycosides are transported across the bacterial cell membrane through **porin** aqueous channels, enter the bacterial cytoplasm, and inhibit protein synthesis by *irreversible* binding of the aminoglycoside to the **30S** bacterial ribosomal subunit (Note: Humans do not have a 30S ribosomal subunit). **The mechanism of resistance is:** plasmid-mediated synthesis of aminoglycoside-inactivating enzymes (e.g., acetyltransferase, phosphotransferase, etc.); modifications of the 30S bacterial ribosomal subunit; and decreased transport of aminoglycosides across the bacterial inner membrane.

   a. **Streptomycin.** Streptomycin is an aminoglycoside that crosses the bacterial outer membrane into the periplasmic space through **aqueous porin channels** and is transported across the bacterial inner membrane by an **oxygen-dependent active transport system,** which is inactivated by Ca^{2+}, Mg^{2+}, low pH, and anaerobic conditions. Streptomycin penetrates tissue fluids well but penetrates tissues and CNS poorly. **Clinical uses include:** Gram-negative aerobic bacilli coverage excellent; tuberculosis caused by *Mycobacterium tuberculosis;* bubonic plague caused by *Yersinia pestis;* tularemia caused by *Francisella tularensis;* brucellosis caused by *Brucella;* bacterial endocarditis caused by group D *Streptococci* and *Streptococcus viridans.*

   b. **Gentamicin (Garamycin), tobramycin (Nebcin), amikacin (Amikin), and netilmicin (Netromycin).** These are similar to streptomycin. **Clinical uses include:** pneumonia caused by *Pseudomonas aeruginosa;* urinary tract infections caused by *Escherichia coli, Enterobacter, Proteus, Klebsiella,* and *Pseudomonas;* bacterial endocarditis caused by group D *Streptococci* and *Streptococcus viridans.*

   c. **Neomycin (Mycifradin) and kanamycin (Kantrex).** These are similar to streptomycin. **Clinical uses include:** bowel sterilization in preparation for surgery; skin infections caused by *Staphylococcus aureus.*

2. **Tetracyclines [tetracycline (Achromycin), doxycycline (Vibramycin), minocycline (Minocin), demeclocycline (Declomycin), oxytetracycline (Terramycin)].** Tetracyclines are a group of related antibiotics that consist of four fused rings with 1–2 conjugated double bonds. **The mechanism of action is:** tetracyclines are transported across the bacterial cell membrane by transport proteins, enter the bacterial cytoplasm, and inhibit protein synthesis by *reversible* binding of tetracycline to the **30S** bacterial ribosomal subunit or by blocking the binding of aminoacyl-transfer RNA (tRNA) to the messenger RNA (mRNA)-ribosome complex. **The mechanism of resistance is:** R-factors that code for an efflux mechanism that pumps tetracyclines out of the bacterial cytoplasm, thereby reducing active tetracycline accumulation within **the bacterial cytoplasm. Clinical uses include:** Gram-positive aerobic and anaerobic coverage excellent; Gram-negative aerobic and anaerobic coverage excellent; pneumonia caused by *Mycoplasma pneumoniae*; Lyme disease caused by *Borrelia burgdorferi*; amebiasis caused by *Entamoeba histolytica*; cholera caused by *Vibrio cholera*; brucellosis caused by *Brucella*; tularemia caused by *Francisella tularensis*; rickettsial diseases (e.g., Rocky Mountain Spotted Fever; Q fever; typhus); chlamydial diseases (e.g., pneumonia, psittacosis, lymphogranuloma venereum); acne; rosacea.

3. **Chloramphenicol [chloramphenicol (Chloromycetin)].** Chloramphenicol contains a nitrobenzene ring and is derived from *Streptomyces venezuelae*. **The mechanism of action is:** chloramphenicol is transported across the bacterial cell membrane by transport proteins, enters the bacterial cytoplasm, and inhibits protein synthesis by *reversible* binding of chloramphenicol to the **50S** bacterial ribosomal subunit, thereby blocking the action of peptidyl transferase, which is responsible for protein elongation. **The mechanism of resistance is:** R-factors that code for acetyl-CoA transferase, which inactivate chloramphenicol. **Clinical uses include:** Gram-positive aerobic and anaerobic coverage excellent; Gram-negative aerobic and anaerobic coverage excellent; meningitis caused by *Haemophilus influenzae*, *Neisseria meningitidis*, and *Streptococcus pneumoniae*; typhoid fever caused by *Salmonella typhi*; rickettsial diseases in children and pregnant women (e.g., Rocky Mountain Spotted Fever; Q fever; typhus); psittacosis caused by *Chlamydia psittaci*; brucellosis caused by *Brucella*; anaerobic infections caused by *Bacteroides*.

4. **Macrolides [erythromycin (E-Mycin, Ilosone, EES, Lactobionate), clarithromycin (Biaxin), azithromycin (Zithromax)].** Macrolides contain a macrocyclic lactone with attached sugars and are derived from *Streptomyces erythreus*. Macrolides are active against intracellular organisms (i.e., they can enter macrophages, neutrophils, and fibroblasts), but have poor penetration of the CNS. **The mechanism of action is:** macrolides are transported across the bacterial cell membrane by transport proteins, enter the bacterial cytoplasm, and inhibit protein synthesis by *reversible* binding of macrolides to the **23S rRNA of the 50S** bacterial ribosomal subunit, thereby blocking translocation of the peptidyl molecule from the A-site to the P-site on mRNA. **The mechanism of resistance is:** plasmids that code for erythromycin esterase, which inactivate macrolides or code for proteins that decrease the transport of macrolides across the bacterial cell membrane; methylation of an adenine residue on the 23S rRNA binding site leading to decreased macrolide affinity for the 50S subunit. **Clinical uses include:** Gram-positive aerobic cocci and bacilli coverage excellent; no Gram-negative coverage; pneumonia caused by *Mycoplasma pneumoniae*; Legionnaires' disease caused by *Legionella pneumophila*; pertussis caused by *Bordetella pertussis*; diphtheria caused by *Corynebacterium diphtheriae*; chancroid caused by *Haemophilus ducreyi*; urethritis caused by *Ureaplasma urealyticum*; tetanus caused by *Clostridium tetani*; gastroenteritis caused by *Campylobacter jejuni*; pneumonia and urogenital infections caused by *Chlamydia*.

5. **Lincosamides [lincomycin (Lincocin), clindamycin (Cleocin)].** Lincosamides are derived from *Streptomyces lincolnensis*. **The mechanism of action is:** lincosamides

are transported across the bacterial cell membrane by transport proteins, enter the bacterial cytoplasm, and inhibit protein synthesis by *reversible* binding of lincosamides to the **23S rRNA of the 50S** bacterial ribosomal subunit, thereby blocking translocation of the peptidyl molecule from the A-site to the P-site on mRNA. **The mechanism of resistance is:** plasmids that code for proteins that decrease the transport of lincosamides across the bacterial cell membrane; methylation of an adenine residue on the 23S rRNA binding site leading to decreased lincosamide affinity for the 50S subunit. **Clinical uses include:** Gram-positive aerobic cocci coverage good; Gram-negative coverage absent; anaerobic coverage good; pneumonia caused by *Pneumocystis carinii*; anaerobic infections caused by *Bacteroides fragilis* and *Clostridium*; acne caused by *Acne vulgaris*.

6. **Oxazolidinones [linezolid (Zyvox)]. The mechanism of action is:** oxazolidinones are transported across the bacterial cell membrane by transport proteins, enter the bacterial cytoplasm, and inhibit protein synthesis by *reversible* binding of oxazolidinones to the **23S rRNA of the 50S** bacterial ribosomal subunit, thereby blocking the formation of the 70S initiation complex. **The mechanism of resistance is:** point mutations in the 23s rRNA leading to decreased oxazolidinone affinity for the 50S subunit. **Clinical uses include:** Gram-positive aerobic cocci and bacilli coverage excellent.

7. **Quinupristin/dalfopristin (Synercid)** is derived from pristamycin. **The mechanism of action is:** Synercid is transported across the bacterial cell membrane by transport proteins, enters the bacterial cytoplasm, and inhibits late and early protein synthesis by binding to bacterial ribosomes. **Clinical uses include:** vancomycin-resistant *Enterococcus faecium* (VREF) bacteremia.

C. DNA replication and transcription inhibitors

1. **Fluoroquinolones [ciprofloxacin (Cipro), ofloxacin (Floxin), norfloxacin (Noroxin)].** Fluoroquinolones are fluorinated analogues of nalidixic acid. **The mechanism of action is:** fluoroquinolones are transported across the bacterial cell membrane by transport proteins, enter the bacterial cytoplasm, and inhibit DNA replication by inhibiting **DNA gyrase** (an enzyme similar to DNA topoisomerase II present in human cells). **The mechanism of resistance is:** plasmids that code for an efflux mechanism that pumps fluoroquinolones out of the bacterial cytoplasm; mutations of bacterial DNA gyrase that reduce the affinity for fluoroquinolones. **Clinical uses include:** Gram-positive aerobic coverage broad; Gram-negative coverage broad; no anaerobic coverage; respiratory infections caused by *Haemophilus influenza*, *Moraxella catarrhalis*, *Streptococcus pneumoniae*, and *Mycoplasma pneumoniae*; nosocomial infections caused by *Pseudomonas aeruginosa*; urinary tract infections caused by *Pseudomonas*, *Klebsiella*, and *Proteus*; chronic bone infections caused by *Pseudomonas* and *Staphylococcus aureus*; gastroenteritis caused by *Escherichia coli*, *Vibrio*, *Shigella*, *Salmonella*, and *Campylobacter jejuni*; sexually transmitted diseases; diabetic foot ulcers; and prostatitis.

2. **Rifampin (Rifadin, Rimactane).** Rifampin is derived from *Streptomyces rifampin* or *Streptomyces mediterranei*. Rifampin penetrates tissues, fluids, and the CNS effectively. **The mechanism of action is:** rifampin is transported across the bacterial cell membrane by transport proteins, enters the bacterial cytoplasm, and inhibits RNA synthesis (i.e., transcription) by inhibiting the **β-subunit of DNA-dependent RNA polymerase. The mechanism of resistance is:** plasmids that code for proteins that reduce transport of rifampin into the bacterial cytoplasm; mutations of bacterial DNA-dependent RNA polymerase that reduce the affinity for rifampin. **Clinical uses include:** Gram-positive coverage good; Gram-negative coverage good; tuberculosis caused by *Mycobacterium tuberculosis*; meningitis caused by *Neisseria meningitidis* or *Haemophilus influenzae*; leprosy caused by *Mycobacterium leprae*; Legionnaires' disease caused by *Legionella pneumophila*; endocarditis and osteomyelitis caused by *Staphylococcus*.

D. **Metabolic inhibitors**

1. **Sulfonamides [sulfisoxazole (Gantrisin), sulfamethoxazole (Gantanol), sulfadiazine, sulfamethizole (Proklar, Thiosulfil), sulfasalazine (Azaline), sulfadoxine, sulfacetamide (Isopto Cetamide), silver sulfadiazine (Silvadene), mafenide (Sulfamylon)].** Sulfonamides are structural analogues of para-aminobenzoic acid (PABA). Sulfonamides cross the placenta (contraindication; pregnancy) and penetrate the CNS effectively. **The mechanism of action is:** sulfonamides are competitive inhibitors of **dihydropteroate synthetase,** which incorporates PABA into dihydropteroic acid in the synthesis of folic acid (Note: Human cells do not make folic acid and are therefore unaffected). The decrease of tetrahydrofolate (THF) inhibits DNA synthesis primarily by decreasing thymidylate synthesis. **The mechanism of resistance is:** bacteria increase the concentration of PABA and thereby out-compete the sulfonamides for dihydropteroate synthetase; R factor-mediated mutations of bacterial dihydropteroate synthetase that reduce the affinity for sulfonamides. **Clinical uses include:** Gram-positive coverage good; Gram-negative coverage good; toxoplasmosis caused by *Toxoplasma gondii*; nocardiosis caused by *Nocardia asteroides*; chancroid caused by *Haemophilus ducreyi*; malaria caused by *Plasmodium falciparum*; urinary tract infections caused by *Escherichia coli* and *Klebsiella*; ocular infections caused by *Chlamydia trachomatis*; burn infection; ulcerative colitis.

2. **Trimethoprim (Trimpex, Proloprim).** Trimethoprim is more potent than the sulfonamides and penetrates tissues, fluids (prostatic and vaginal), and the CNS effectively. **The mechanism of action is:** trimethoprim is a competitive inhibitor of **dihydrofolate reductase,** which coverts dihydrofolate (DHF) to THF in the synthesis of folic acid (Note: Human cells do not make folic acid and are therefore unaffected). The decrease of THF inhibits DNA synthesis primarily by decreasing thymidylate synthesis. **The mechanism of resistance is:** R factor-mediated mutations of bacterial **dihydrofolate reductase** that reduce the affinity for trimethoprim.

3. **Trimethoprim/sulfamethoxazole (Bactrim, Septra, TMP-SMX).** These two drugs are usually combined so that the synergistic effect inhibits folic acid synthesis at two steps. This combination has the advantages of increased potency, increased spectrum of coverage, and a decreased incidence of resistance. **Clinical uses include:** Gram-positive coverage good; Gram-negative coverage good; pneumonia caused by *Pneumocystis carinii*; acute otitis media, acute chronic bronchitis, and acute maxillary sinusitis caused by *Haemophilus influenzae* and *Streptococcus pneumoniae*; nocardiosis caused by *Nocardia asteroides*; chancroid caused by *Haemophilus ducreyi*; shigellosis caused by *Shigella*; typhoid fever caused by *Salmonella typhi*; urinary tract infections caused by *Escherichia coli*, *Proteus*, and *Klebsiella*; gonorrhea; bacterial prostatitis.

IV Antimycobacterial Drugs

Mycobacterium tuberculosis causes tuberculosis (TB), which is the classic mycobacterial disease. Aerosolized infectious particles travel to terminal airways, where *Mycobacterium tuberculosis* penetrates unactivated alveolar macrophages and **inhibits acidification of endolysosomes** so that alveolar macrophages cannot kill the bacteria. However, replicating intracellular *Mycobacterium tuberculosis* stimulates CD8+ cytotoxic T cells, which lyse infected cells and CD4+ helper T cells, which release interferon-γ and other cytokines that activate macrophages to phagocytose and kill the bacteria. The **Ghon complex** is the first lesion of primary TB and consists of a **parenchymal granuloma** (location is **subpleural** and in **lower lobes of the lung**) and **prominent, infected mediastinal lymph nodes.** Most cases of primary TB are asymptomatic and resolve spontaneously. TB is treated with multiple drug regimens, which include:

A. **Rifampin (Rifadin, Rimactane).** Rifampin is derived from *Streptomyces rifampin* or *Streptomyces mediterranei*. Rifampin penetrates tissues, fluids, and the CNS effectively. **The mechanism of action is:** rifampin is transported across the bacterial cell membrane by transport proteins, enters the bacterial cytoplasm, and inhibits RNA synthesis (i.e., transcription) by inhibiting the β-subunit of DNA-dependent RNA polymerase. **The mechanism of resistance is:** plasmids that code for proteins that reduce transport of rifampin into the bacterial cytoplasm; mutations of bacterial DNA-dependent RNA polymerase that reduce the affinity for rifampin. **Clinical uses include:** Gram-positive coverage good; Gram-negative coverage good; tuberculosis caused by *Mycobacterium tuberculosis*; meningitis caused by *Neisseria meningitidis* or *Haemophilus influenzae*; leprosy caused by *Mycobacterium leprae*; Legionnaires' disease caused by *Legionella pneumophila*; endocarditis and osteomyelitis caused by *Staphylococcus*.

B. Isoniazid (Laniazid). Isoniazid penetrates tissues, fluids, and the CNS effectively. Isoniazid is the only drug used as a solo prophylactic agent, although it is primarily used in combination with other drugs. Isoniazid is the most important antimycobacterial drug against TB worldwide. **The mechanism of action is:** inhibition of mycolic acid synthesis, which are important components of the cell wall.

C. Pyrazinamide. The mechanism of action is unknown.

D. Ethambutol (Myambutol). The mechanism of action is unknown.

E. Streptomycin. Streptomycin is an aminoglycoside that crosses the bacterial outer membrane into the periplasmic space through **aqueous porin channels** and is transported across the bacterial inner membrane by an **oxygen-dependent active transport system,** which is inactivated by Ca^{2+}, Mg^{2+}, low pH, and anaerobic conditions. Streptomycin penetrates tissue fluids well but penetrates tissues and CNS poorly. **The mechanism of action is:** inhibition of protein synthesis by *irreversible* binding of the aminoglycoside to the **30S** bacterial ribosomal subunit. (Note: Humans do not have a 30S ribosomal subunit.)

Antifungal Drugs

Fungi cause infections called **mycoses.** The cell membranes of fungi contain **ergosterol** while the cell membranes of human cells contain cholesterol.

A. Polyene antifungal agents
1. **Amphotericin-B (Fungizone). The mechanism of action is:** binds ergosterol and punches holes in the fungal cell membrane, which increases cell permeability and results in fungal cell death by osmotic disruption. **Clinical uses include:** histoplasmosis caused by *Histoplasma capsulatum*; coccidioidomycosis caused by *Coccidioides immitis*; blastomycosis caused by *Blastomyces dermatitidis*; aspergillosis caused by *Aspergillus fumingatus*; cryptococcosis caused by *Cryptococcus neoformans*; and systemic candidiasis.
2. **Nystatin (Mycostatin). The mechanism of action is:** binds ergosterol and punches holes in the fungal cell membrane, which increases cell permeability and results in fungal cell death by osmotic disruption. **Clinical uses include:** oral, esophageal, or vaginal candidiasis.

B. Azoles
1. **Ketoconazole (Nizoral).** Ketoconazole does not penetrate the CNS effectively. **The mechanism of action is:** inhibits cytochrome P_{450} enzymes, which blocks ergosterol synthesis needed for the fungal cell membrane and results in fungal cell death by osmotic disruption. **Clinical uses include:** histoplasmosis caused by *Histoplasma capsulatum*; coccidioidomycosis caused by *Coccidioides immitis*; blastomycosis caused by *Blastomyces dermatitidis*; and oropharyngeal candidiasis.
2. **Fluconazole (Diflucan).** Fluconazole penetrates the CNS effectively. **The mechanism of action is:** inhibits cytochrome P_{450} enzymes, which block ergosterol synthesis needed for the fungal cell membrane and results in fungal cell death by osmotic disruption. **Clinical uses include:** histoplasmosis caused by *Histoplasma*

capsulatum; coccidioidomycosis caused by *Coccidioides immitis;* blastomycosis caused by *Blastomyces dermatitidis;* and oropharyngeal candidiasis.

3. **Itraconazole (Sporanox).** Itraconazole requires acid pH for absorption. **The mechanism of action is:** inhibits cytochrome P$_{450}$ enzymes, which block ergosterol synthesis needed for the fungal cell membrane and results in fungal cell death by osmotic disruption. **Clinical uses include:** histoplasmosis caused by *Histoplasma capsulatum;* coccidioidomycosis caused by *Coccidioides immitis;* blastomycosis caused by *Blastomyces dermatitidis;* aspergillosis caused by *Aspergillus fumingatus;* cryptococcosis caused by *Cryptococcus neoformans;* mucocutaneous candidiasis; tinea infections.

4. **Miconazole (Monistat) and clotrimazole. The mechanism of action is:** inhibits cytochrome P$_{450}$ enzymes, which block ergosterol synthesis needed for the fungal cell membrane and results in fungal cell death by osmotic disruption. **Clinical uses include:** commonly used for topical fungal infections.

5. **Flucytosine (Ancobon). The mechanism of action is: flucytosine** is converted to 5′fluoro-uridine monophosphate (5F-UMP), which inhibits thymidylate synthetase and prevents the formation of deoxythymidine monophosphate (dTMP). **Clinical uses include:** cryptococcal infections and candidiasis.

6. **Griseofulvin (Fulvicin). The mechanism of action is:** inhibits mitosis by binding to tubulin, which disrupts microtubule formation and arrests cells in metaphase of the cell cycle. **Clinical uses include:** dermatophytic infections only of the skin, hair, and nails.

Ⅵ Antiviral Drugs

A. Antiherpetic drugs. These drugs are used against the herpes viruses, which are **linear, double-stranded, encapsulated DNA viruses.**

1. **Acyclovir (Avirax, Zovirax).** Acyclovir (Acy) is a **guanine analogue,** which is converted to Acy monophosphate (AcyMP) by thymidylate kinase encoded by the herpes simplex virus. AcyMP is then converted to Acy diphosphate (AcyDP) and Acy triphosphate (AcyTP) by cellular enzymes. **The mechanism of action is:** inhibits viral DNA replication because AcyTP disrupts the action of viral DNA polymerase. **Clinical uses include:** mucocutaneous herpes, genital herpes, herpes encephalitis caused by herpes simplex type I and II; varicella (chickenpox), zoster (shingles), and herpes zoster ophthalmicus caused by varicella zoster virus. Acyclovir is not effective against cytomegalovirus (CMV) or Epstein-Barr virus (EBV).

2. **Ganciclovir (Cytovene).** Ganciclovir (Gan) is a **guanine analogue,** which is converted to Gan triphosphate (GanTP). **The mechanism of action is:** inhibits viral DNA replication because GanTP disrupts the action of viral DNA polymerase. **Clinical uses include:** CMV infections.

3. **Idoxuridine (Stoxil).** Idoxuridine (Ido) is a **thymidine analogue,** which is converted to Ido triphosphate (IdoTP) by cellular enzymes. **The mechanism of action is:** inhibits viral DNA replication because IdoTP disrupts the action of viral DNA polymerase. **Clinical uses include:** keratitis caused by herpes simplex virus or vaccinia virus.

4. **Vidarabine (Vira-A).** Vidarabine (Vid) is an **adenosine analogue,** which is converted to Vid triphosphate (VidTP) by cellular enzymes. **The mechanism of action is:** inhibits viral DNA replication because VidTP disrupts the action of viral DNA polymerase. **Clinical uses include:** keratoconjunctivitis and encephalitis caused by herpes simplex virus.

5. **Foscarnet (Foscavir).** Foscarnet is a phosphonoformate derivative that does not require phosphorylation. **The mechanism of action is:** inhibits viral DNA replication by blocking the pyrophosphate-binding site of viral DNA polymerase. **Clinical uses include:** CMV retinitis in AIDS patients; acyclovir-resistant strains of herpes virus in AIDS patients.

B. **Antiretroviral drugs.** These drugs are used against retroviruses, which are **single-stranded, positive-sense RNA (ss+RNA) viruses.** These viruses encode a **reverse transcriptase (also called RNA-dependent DNA polymerase)** and replicate through a **DNA intermediate.**

1. **Didanosine (Dideoxyinosine, ddI, Videx).** Didanosine (Did) is an **adenosine analogue,** which is converted to Did triphosphate (DidTP) by cellular enzymes. **The mechanism of action is:** inhibits the replication of the viral DNA intermediate because DidTP disrupts the action of viral reverse transcriptase and terminates elongation of the viral DNA intermediate. **Clinical uses include:** HIV-infected patients.

2. **Zalcitabine (Dideoxycytidine, ddC, HIVID).** Zalcitabine (Zal) is a **cytosine analogue,** which is converted to Zal triphosphate (ZalTP) by cellular enzymes. **The mechanism of action is:** inhibits the replication of the viral DNA intermediate because ZalTP disrupts the action of viral reverse transcriptase and terminates elongation of the viral DNA intermediate. **Clinical uses include:** advanced HIV-infected patients.

3. **Zidovudine (AZT, Retrovir).** Zidovudine (Zid) is a **thymidine analogue,** which is converted to Zid triphosphate (ZidTP) by cellular enzymes. **The mechanism of action is:** inhibits the replication of the viral DNA intermediate because ZidTP disrupts the action of viral reverse transcriptase and terminates elongation of the viral DNA intermediate. **Clinical uses include:** HIV-infected patients.

C. **Other antiviral drugs.** These drugs are mainly used against influenza type A and respiratory syncytial virus (RSV), which are **single-stranded, negative-sense RNA (ss-RNA) viruses.**

1. **Ribavirin (Virazole).** Ribavirin is a **guanosine analogue. The mechanism of action is:** reduces the guanosine triphosphate (GTP) pools and inhibits viral RNA replication and viral protein synthesis. **Clinical uses include:** RSV.

2. **Amantadine (Symmetrel), rimantadine (Flumadine). The mechanism of action is:** inhibits viral uncoating of influenza virus type A by blocking the action of the M_2 membrane protein, which pumps H^+ into the endolysosome, lowers the pH, and promotes viral uncoating. **Clinical uses include:** influenza caused by influenza virus type A in young, elderly, and immunosuppressed individuals.

VII   Summary Table of Drugs *(Table 8-1)*

TABLE 8-1	SUMMARY TABLE OF DRUGS
Drug Class	**Drug**
Antiasthmatic drugs	**β_2–adrenergic agonists:** terbutaline, albuterol, metaproterenol, and salmeterol **M₃AChR antagonists:** atropine and ipratropium, cromolyn (NasalCrom) **Corticosteroids:** beclomethasone, budesonide, triamcinolone
Allergy, hay fever, rhinitis, and urticaria drugs	**1st generation H₁–receptor antagonists:** diphenhydramine (Benadryl), dimenhydrinate (Dramamine), chlorpheniramine (Chlor-Trimeton), and meclizine (Antivert) **2nd generation H₁–receptor antagonists:** fexofenadine (Allegra), desloratadine (Clarinex), and cetirizine (Zyrtec)

TABLE 8-1	SUMMARY TABLE OF DRUGS (*CONTINUED*)

Drug Class	Drug
Antibiotics	**Cell wall synthesis inhibitors** **Natural penicillins:** penicillin G (Pfizerpen), penicillin V (V-Cillin K), penicillin G procaine (Duracillin A.S.), penicillin G benzathine (Bicillin L-A) **Anti-staphylococcal penicillins:** methicillin (Staphcillin), nafcillin (Unipen), oxacillin (Bactocill), DICLOXACILLIN (Dynapen), cloxacillin (Tegopen) **Aminopenicillins:** ampicillin (Omnipen), amoxicillin (Amoxil) **Antipseudomonal penicillins:** mezlocillin (Mezlin), piperacillin (Pipracil), azlocillin (Azlin), carbenicillin (Geopen), ticarcillin (Ticar) **1st generation cephalosporins:** cephalothin (Keflin), cephapirin (Cefadyl), cephradine (Velosef), cephalexin (Keflex), cefazolin (Ancef), cefadroxil (Duricef) **2nd generation cephalosporins:** cefamandole (Mandol), cefaclor (Ceclor), cefoxitin (Mefoxin), cefotetan (Cefotan), cefonicid (Monocid), cefprozil (Cefzil), cefuroxime (Ceftin), cefpodoxime proxetil (Vantin) **3rd generation cephalosporins:** ceftriaxone (Rocephin), ceftazidime (Fortaz), cefotaxime (Claforan), ceftizoxime (Cefizox), moxalactam (Moxam), cefixime (Suprax), cefoperazone (Cefobid), imipenem/cilastatin (Primaxin), aztreonam (Azactam), vancomycin (Vancocin), cycloserine (Seromycin) **β-lactamase inhibitors:** clavulanic acid (Augmentin), sulbactam (Unasyn), tazobactam cefepime (Maxipime) **Protein synthesis inhibitors** **Aminoglycosides:** streptomycin, gentamicin (Garamycin), tobramycin (Nebcin), amikacin (Amikin), netilmicin (Netromycin), neomycin (Mycifradin), kanamycin (Kantrex) **Tetracyclines:** tetracycline (Achromycin), doxycycline (Vibramycin), minocycline (Minocin), demeclocycline (Declomycin), oxytetracycline (Terramycin), chloramphenicol (Chloromycetin) **Macrolides:** erythromycin (E-Mycin, Ilosone, EES, Lactobionate), clarithromycin (Biaxin), azithromycin (Zithromax) **Lincosamides:** lincomycin (Lincocin), clindamycin (Cleocin) **Oxazolidinones:** linezolid (Zyvox), quinupristin/dalfopristin (Synercid) **DNA replication and transcription inhibitors** **Fluoroquinolones:** ciprofloxacin (Cipro), ofloxacin (Floxin), norfloxacin (Noroxin), rifampin (Rifadin, Rimactane) **Metabolic Inhibitors** **Sulfonamides:** sulfisoxazole (Gantrisin), sulfamethoxazole (Gantanol), sulfadiazine, sulfamethizole (Proklar, Thiosulfil), sulfasalazine (Azaline), sulfadoxine, sulfacetamide (Isopto Cetamide), silver sulfadiazine (Silvadene), mafenide (Sulfamylon), trimethoprim (Trimpex, Proloprim), trimethoprim/sulfamethoxazole (Bactrim, Septra, TMP-SMX)
Antimycobacterial drugs	Rifampin (Rifadin, Rimactane) Isoniazid (Laniazid) Pyrazinamide Ethambutol (Myambutol) Streptomycin
Antifungal Drugs	**Polyene agents:** amphotericin-B (Fungizone), nystatin (Mycostatin) **Azoles:** ketoconazole (Nizoral), fluconazole (Diflucan), itraconazole (Sporanox), miconazole (Monistat) and clotrimazole, flucytosine (Ancobon), griseofulvin (Fulvicin)
Antiviral drugs **Antiherpetic drugs**	**Guanine analogue:** Acyclovir (Avirax, Zovirax), ganciclovir (Cytovene) **Thymidine analogue:** idoxuridine (Stoxil)
Antiretroviral drugs	**Adenosine analogue:** vidarabine (Vira-A), foscarnet (Foscavir) **Adenosine analogue:** didanosine (Dideoxyinosine, ddI, Videx) **Cytosine analogue:** zalcitabine (Dideoxycytidine, ddC, HIVID) **Thymidine analogue:** zidovudine (AZT, Retrovir)
Other Viral Drugs	**Guanosine analogue:** ribavirin (Virazole), amantadine (Symmetrel), rimantadine (Flumadine)

Credits

Figure 1-1: **A, B, C** From Dudek RW. High-Yield Embryology, 2nd ed. Philadelphia: LWW, 2001, page 56. **D, E, F, G, H** From Yamada T, et al. Textbook of Gastroenterology, vol 1, 3rd ed. Philadelphia: LWW, 1999, page 1186. **D-1** From Kirks DR. Radiograph: Practical Pediatric Imaging, 3rd ed. Philadelphia: LWW, 1998, page 845. **F-1** From Avery GB, et al. Radiograph: Neonatology: Pathophysiology and Management of the Newborn, 5th ed. Philadelphia: LWW, 1999, page 1018. **I** From Kirks DR. Practical Pediatric Imaging, 3rd ed. Philadelphia: LWW, 1998, page 662. **J** From Kirks DR. Practical Pediatric Imaging, 3rd ed. Philadelphia: LWW, 1998, page 663. **K** From Swischuk LE. Imaging of the Newborn, Infant, and Young Child, 5th ed. Philadelphia: LWW, 2004, page 101.

Figure 1-2: **A** From Rohen JW. Color Atlas of Anatomy, 4th ed. Baltimore: LWW, 1998, page 235. **B** From Kirks DR. Practical Pediatric Imaging, 3rd ed. Philadelphia: LWW, 1998, page 671. **C** From Kirks DR. Practical Pediatric Imaging, 3rd ed. Philadelphia: LWW, 1998, page 674. **D** From Swischuk LE. Imaging of the Newborn, Infant, and Young Child, 5th ed. Philadelphia: LWW, 2004, page 161. **E** From Kirks DR. Practical Pediatric Imaging, 3rd ed. Philadelphia: LWW, 1998, page 676. Courtesy of Kenneth Hawkins, MD, Birmingham, AL. **F** From Kirks DR. Practical Pediatric Imaging, 3rd ed. Philadelphia: LWW, 1998, page 676. **G** From Kirks DR. Practical Pediatric Imaging, 3rd ed. Philadelphia: LWW, 1998, page 679.

Figure 1-3: **(1), (2), (3), (4)** Modified from Rohen JW. Color Atlas of Anatomy, 4th ed. Baltimore: LWW, 1998, page 235. **A, B, C** Adapted from Sweeny LJ. Basic Concepts in Embryology. New York: McGraw Hill, 1998, page 321. **D** From Ross MH, Kaye GI, Pawlina W. Histology A Text and Atlas, 4th ed. Baltimore: LWW, 2003, page 599.

Figure 1-4: **A** From Swischuk LE. Imaging of the Newborn, Infant, and Young Child, 5th ed. Philadelphia: LWW, 2004, page 39. **B** From Dudek RW. High-Yield Embryology, 2nd ed. Philadelphia: LWW, 2001, page 59. **C** From Kirks DR. Practical Pediatric Imaging, 3rd ed. Philadelphia: LWW, 1998, page 695. **D** From Avery GB, et al. Radiograph: Neonatology: Pathophysiology and Management of the Newborn, 5th ed. Philadelphia: LWW, 1999, page 518. **E** From Swischuk LE. Imaging of the Newborn, Infant, and Young Child, 5th ed. Philadelphia: LWW, 2004, page 51. **F** From Swischuk LE. Imaging of the Newborn, Infant, and Young Child, 5th ed. Philadelphia: LWW, 2004, page 37. **G** From Avery GB, et al. Radiograph: Neonatology: Pathophysiology and Management of the Newborn, 5th ed. Philadelphia: LWW, 1999, page 507. **H** From Swischuk LE. Imaging of the Newborn, Infant, and Young Child, 5th ed. Philadelphia: LWW, 2004, page 76. **I** From Swischuk LE. Imaging of the Newborn, Infant, and Young Child, 5th ed. Philadelphia: LWW, 2004, page 61. **J** From Swischuk LE. Imaging of the Newborn, Infant, and Young Child, 5th ed. Philadelphia: LWW, 2004, page 59. **K** From Swischuk LE. Imaging of the Newborn, Infant, and Young Child, 5th ed. Philadelphia: LWW, 2004, page 69. **L** From Swischuk LE. Imaging of the Newborn, Infant, and Young Child, 5th ed. Philadelphia: LWW, 2004, page 42.

Figure 1-5: **A** From Kirks DR. Practical Pediatric Imaging, 3rd ed. Philadelphia: LWW, 1998, page 669. **B** From Kirks DR. Practical Pediatric Imaging, 3rd ed. Philadelphia: LWW, 1998, page 683. **C** From Swischuk LE. Imaging of the Newborn, Infant, and Young Child, 5th ed. Philadelphia: LWW, 2004, page 64. **D** Redrawn and modified from Dudek RW. High-Yield Embryology, 2nd ed. Philadelphia: LWW, 2001, page 24.

Figure 1-6: **A** From Kirks DR. Practical Pediatric Imaging, 3rd ed. Philadelphia: LWW, 1998, page 630. **B** From Kirks DR. Practical Pediatric Imaging, 3rd ed. Philadelphia: LWW, 1998, page 630. **C** From Kirks DR. Practical Pediatric Imaging, 3rd ed. Philadelphia: LWW, 1998, page 631. **D** From Swischuk LE. Imaging of the Newborn, Infant, and Young Child, 5th ed. Philadelphia: LWW, 2004, page 6. **E** From Swischuk LE. Imaging of the Newborn, Infant, and Young Child, 5th ed. Philadelphia: LWW, 2004, page 4.

Figure 2-1: **A** From Dudek RW. High-Yield Gross Anatomy, 2nd ed. Baltimore: LWW, 2002, page 24. **B** From Brandt WE, Helms CA. Fundamentals of Diagnostic Radiology, 2nd ed. Baltimore: LWW, 1999, page 496. **C** From Brandt WE, Helms CA. Fundamentals of Diagnostic Radiology, 2nd ed. Baltimore: LWW, 1999, page 496. **D** From Daffner RH. Clinical Radiology: The Essentials, 2nd ed. Baltimore: LWW, 1999, page 243. **E** From Daffner RH. Clinical Radiology: The Essentials, 2nd ed. Baltimore: LWW, 1999, page 245.

Figure 2-2: **A** From Dudek RW. High-Yield Gross Anatomy, 2nd ed. Baltimore: LWW, 2002, page 27. **B** From Swischuk LE. Imaging of the Newborn, Infant, and Young Child, 5th ed. Philadelphia: LWW, 2004, page 288. **C** From Brandt WE, Helms CA. Fundamentals of Diagnostic Radiology, 2nd ed. Baltimore: LWW, 1999, page 579. **D** From Brandt WE, Helms CA. Fundamentals of Diagnostic Radiology, 2nd ed. Baltimore: LWW, 1999, page 582. **E** From Brandt WE, Helms CA. Fundamentals of Diagnostic Radiology, 2nd ed. Baltimore: LWW, 1999, page 596.

Figure 2-3: **A** From Dudek RW. High-Yield Gross Anatomy, 2nd ed. Baltimore: LWW, 2002, page 29. Adapted with permission from Moore KL. Clinically Oriented Anatomy, 3rd ed. Baltimore: LWW, 1992, page 57. **Inset** Adapted with permission from Chen H, Sonneday CJ, Lillemoe KD, eds. Manual of Common Bedside Surgical Procedures, 2nd ed. Philadelphia: LWW, 2000, page 123. **B** Adapted from Moore KL. Clinically Oriented Anatomy, 3rd ed. Baltimore: LWW, 1992, page 213. **C** From Dudek RW. High-Yield Gross Anatomy, 2nd ed. Baltimore: LWW, 2002, page 30. **D** From Daffner RH. Clinical Radiology: The Essentials, 2nd ed. Baltimore: LWW, 1999, page 93.

Figure 2-4: **A** From Brandt WE, Helms CA. Fundamentals of Diagnostic Radiology, 2nd ed. Baltimore: LWW, 1999, page 463. **B** From Dudek RW. High-Yield Gross Anatomy 2nd ed. Baltimore: LWW, 2002, page 36. Adapted with permission from Freundlich IM, Bragg DG. A Radiologic Approach to Diseases of the Chest, 2nd ed. Baltimore: LWW, 1997, page 270.

Figure 2-5: **A** From Rohen JW. Color Atlas of Anatomy, 4th ed. Baltimore: LWW, 1998, page 235. **B, C** Adapted from Collins J, Stern EJ. Chest Radiology: The Essentials. Philadelphia: LWW, 1999, pages 10 and 11.

Figure 3-1: From Collins J, Stern EJ. Chest Radiology: The Essentials. Philadelphia: LWW, 1999, page 3.

Figure 3-2: From Collins J, Stern EJ. Chest Radiology: The Essentials. Philadelphia: LWW, 1999, page 4.

Figure 3-3: From Collins J, Stern EJ. Chest Radiology: The Essentials. Philadelphia: LWW, 1999, page 5.

Figure 3-4: Modified and reprinted from Collins J, Stern EJ. Chest Radiology: The Essentials. Philadelphia: LWW, 1999, page 5.

Figure 3-5: Modified and reprinted from Collins J, Stern EJ. Chest Radiology: The Essentials. Philadelphia: LWW, 1999, page 5.

Figure 3-6: From Slaby F, Jacobs ER. Radiographic Anatomy, NMS Series. Philadelphia: Harwal, 1990, page 108.

Figure 3-7: **A** From Slaby F, Jacobs ER. Radiographic Anatomy, NMS Series. Philadelphia: Harwal, 1990, page 110. **B** From Barret CP, Andersen LD, Holder LE, Pliakoff SJ. Primer of Sectional Anatomy with MRI and CT Correlation, 2nd ed. Baltimore: LWW, 1994, page 54.

Figure 3-8: **A** From Slaby F, Jacobs ER. Radiographic Anatomy, NMS Series. Philadelphia: Harwal, 1990, page 112. **B** From Barret CP, Andersen LD, Holder LE, Pliakoff SJ. Primer of Sectional Anatomy with MRI and CT Correlation, 2nd ed. Baltimore: LWW, 1994, page 56.

Figure 3-9: **A** From Slaby F, Jacobs ER. Radiographic Anatomy, NMS Series. Philadelphia: Harwal, 1990, page 116.

Figure 3-10: **A** From Slaby F, Jacobs ER. Radiographic Anatomy, NMS Series. Philadelphia: Harwal, 1990, page 118. **B** From Barret CP, Andersen LD, Holder LE, Pliakoff SJ. Primer of Sectional Anatomy with MRI and CT Correlation, 2nd ed. Baltimore: LWW, 1994, page 60.

Figure 3-11: **A** From Slaby F, Jacobs ER. Radiographic Anatomy, NMS Series. Philadelphia: Harwal, 1990, page 118. **B** From Barret CP, Andersen LD, Holder LE, Pliakoff SJ. Primer of Sectional Anatomy with MRI and CT Correlation, 2nd ed. Baltimore: LWW, 1994, page 62.

Figure 4-1: Modified from Rohen JW. Color Atlas of Anatomy, 4th ed. Baltimore: LWW, 1998, page 235.

Figure 4-2: **A** From Cormack DH. Essential Histology, 2nd ed. Baltimore: LWW, 2001, Plate 14-1. **B** From Cormack DH. Essential Histology, 2nd ed. Baltimore: LWW, 2001, Plate 14-2. **C** From Sternberg SS. Histology for Pathologists, 2nd ed. Baltimore: LWW, 1997, page 436. **D** From Copenhaver WM, Bunge RP, Bunge MB. Bailey's Textbook of Histology, 16th ed. Philadelphia: LWW, 1971, page 508.

Figure 4-3: **A** From Sternberg SS. Histology for Pathologists, 2nd ed. Baltimore: LWW, 1997, page 437. **B and inset** Courtesy of E. R. Weibel, MD. **C** From Sternberg SS. Histology for Pathologists, 2nd ed. Baltimore: LWW, 1997, page 439. **D** From Takamura T, Rom WN, Ferrans VJ, Crystal RG. Morphological Characterization of Alveolar Macrophages from Subjects with Occupational Exposure to Inorganic Particles. Am Rev Respir Dis 1989;140:1674–1685.

Figure 4-4: **A** From Zeltner TB, Burri PH. The Postnatal Development and Growth of the Human Lung. II. Morphology Respir Physiol 1987;67:269–282. **B** From Cormack DH. Essential Histology, 2nd ed. Baltimore: LWW, 2001, page 345. **C** From Cormack DH. Essential Histology, 2nd ed. Baltimore: LWW, 2001, page 345. Courtesy of E. R. Weibel, MD. **D** From Dudek RW. High-Yield Histology, 3rd ed. Baltimore: LWW, 2004, page 171. Originally from Ross MH, Kaye GI, Pawlina W. Histology A Text and Atlas, 4th ed. Baltimore: LWW, 2003, page 587.

Figure 5-6: **Top** Modified from Rohen JW. Color Atlas of Anatomy, 4th ed. Baltimore: LWW, 1998, page 235. **Bottom** From Cormack DH. Essential Histology, 2nd ed. Baltimore: LWW, 2001, page 345. Courtesy of E. R. Weibel, MD.

Figure 5-8: Modified from Dudek RW. High-Yield Histology, 2nd ed. Baltimore: LWW, 2000, page 80.

Figure 6-2: **A** From Collins J, Stern EJ. Chest Radiology: The Essentials. Philadelphia: LWW, 1999, page 171. **B** From Dudek RW. High-Yield Embryology, 2nd ed. Baltimore: LWW, 2001, page 59. **C** From Collins J, Stern EJ. Chest Radiology: The Essentials. Philadelphia: LWW, 1999, page 50. **D** From Damjanov I. Histopathology: A Color Atlas and Textbook. Baltimore: LWW, 1996, page 131. **E** From Collins J, Stern EJ. Chest Radiology: The Essentials. Philadelphia: LWW, 1999, page 183. **F** From Daffner RH. Clinical Radiology: The Essentials, 2nd ed. Baltimore: LWW, 1999, page 158. **G** From Collins J, Stern EJ. Chest Radiology: The Essentials. Philadelphia: LWW, 1999, page 195. **H** From Freundlich IM, Bragg DG. A Radiologic Approach to Diseases of the Chest, 2nd ed. Baltimore: LWW, 1997, page 716.

Figure 6-3: **A** From Daffner RH. Clinical Radiology: The Essentials, 2nd ed. Baltimore: LWW, 1999, page 146. **B** From Damjanov I. Histopathology: A Color Atlas and Textbook. Baltimore: LWW, 1996, page 141. **C** Redrawn from West JB. Pulmonary Pathophysiology: The Essentials, 5th ed. Baltimore: LWW, 1998, page 53. **D** From Rubin E, Farber JL. Pathology, 3rd ed. Baltimore: LWW, 1999, page 629. **F** From Damjanov I. Histopathology: A Color Atlas and Textbook. Baltimore: LWW, 1996, page 144.

Figure 6-4: **A** From Daffner RH. Clinical Radiology: The Essentials, 2nd ed. Baltimore: LWW, 1999, page 152. **B** From Sternberg SS. Diagnostic Surgical Pathology, vol 1, 3rd ed. Baltimore: LWW, 1999, page 1013. **C** From Rubin E, Farber JL. Pathology, 3rd ed. Baltimore: LWW, 1999, page 637. **D** From Damjanov I. Histopathology: A Color Atlas and Textbook. Baltimore: LWW, 1996, page 143. **E** From Rubin E, Farber JL. Pathology, 3rd ed. Baltimore: LWW, 1999, page 634. **F** From Rubin E, Farber JL. Pathology, 3rd ed. Baltimore: LWW, 1999, page 636. **G** From Rubin E, Farber JL. Pathology, 3rd ed. Baltimore: LWW, 1999, page 634. **H** From Damjanov I. Histopathology: A Color Atlas and Textbook. Baltimore: LWW, 1996, page 143. **I** From Sternberg SS. Diagnostic Surgical Pathology, vol 1, 3rd ed. Baltimore: LWW, 1999, page 1055. **J** From Sternberg SS. Histology for Pathologists, 2nd ed. Baltimore: LWW, 1997, page 452. **K** From Sternberg SS. Histology for Pathologists, 2nd ed. Baltimore: LWW, 1997, page 452.

Figure 6-5: **A** From Collins J, Stern EJ. Chest Radiology: The Essentials. Philadelphia: LWW, 1999, page 94. **B** From Collins J, Stern EJ. Chest Radiology: The Essentials. Philadelphia: LWW, 1999, page 94. **C** From Sternberg SS. Diagnostic Surgical Pathology, vol 1, 3rd ed. Baltimore: LWW, 1999, page 1086.

D From Sternberg SS. Diagnostic Surgical Pathology, vol 1, 3rd ed. Baltimore: LWW, 1999, page 1086. **E** From Sternberg SS. Diagnostic Surgical Pathology, vol 1, 3rd ed. Baltimore: LWW, 1999, page 1085. **F** From Sternberg SS. Diagnostic Surgical Pathology, vol 1, 3rd ed. Baltimore: LWW, 1999, page 1085. **G** From Cagle PT. Color Atlas and Text of Pulmonary Pathology. Philadelphia: LWW, 2005. **H** From Sternberg SS. Diagnostic Surgical Pathology, vol 1, 3rd ed. Baltimore: LWW, 1999, page 1080. **I** From Sternberg SS. Diagnostic Surgical Pathology, vol 1, 3rd ed. Baltimore: LWW, 1999, page 1093. **J** From Sternberg SS. Diagnostic Surgical Pathology, vol 1, 3rd ed. Baltimore: LWW, 1999, page 1096.

Figure 6-6: **A** From Freundlich IM, Bragg DG. A Radiologic Approach to Diseases of the Chest, 2nd ed. Baltimore: LWW, 1997, page 309. **B** Courtesy of R. W. Dudek, Ph.D. Dudek RW. High-Yield Histology, 2nd ed. Baltimore: LWW, 2000, page 135.

Figure 7-1: **A** Modified and redrawn from Rubin E, Farber JL. Pathology, 3rd ed. Baltimore: LWW, 1999, page 603. **B** Modified and redrawn from Rubin E, Farber JL. Pathology, 3rd ed. Baltimore: LWW, 1999, page 612. **A-1** From Damjanov I. Histopathology: A Color Atlas and Textbook. Baltimore: LWW, 1996, page 133. **B-1** From Damjanov I. Histopathology: A Color Atlas and Textbook. Baltimore: LWW, 1996, page 135.

Figure 7-2: **A** From Brandt WE, Helms CA. Fundamentals of Diagnostic Radiology, 2nd ed. Baltimore: LWW, 1999, page 402. **B** From Burton GRW, Engelkird PG. Microbiology for the Health Sciences, 7th ed. Baltimore: LWW, 2004, page 1. **C** From Koneman EW, et al. Color Atlas and Textbook of Diagnostic Microbiology, 5th ed. Baltimore: LWW, 1997, Color Plate 12-1C. **D** From Koneman EW, et al. Color Atlas and Textbook of Diagnostic Microbiology, 5th ed. Baltimore: LWW, 1997, Color Plate 12-1D. **E** From Koneman EW, et al. Color Atlas and Textbook of Diagnostic Microbiology, 5th ed. Baltimore: LWW, 1997, Color Plate 12-3A. **F** From Koneman EW, et al. Color Atlas and Textbook of Diagnostic Microbiology, 5th ed. Baltimore: LWW, 1997, Color Plate 12-3B.

Figure 7-3: **A** From Collins J, Stern EJ. Chest Radiology: The Essentials. Philadelphia: LWW, 1999, page 103. **B** From Burton GRW, Engelkird PG. Microbiology for the Health Sciences, 7th ed. Baltimore: LWW, 2004, page 2. **C** From Burton GRW, Engelkird PG. Microbiology for the Health Sciences, 7th ed. Baltimore: LWW, 2004. **D** From Koneman EW, et al. Color Atlas and Textbook of Diagnostic Microbiology, 5th ed. Baltimore: LWW, 1997, Color Plate 11-1D. **E** From Koneman EW, et al. Color Atlas and Textbook of Diagnostic Microbiology, 5th ed. Baltimore: LWW, 1997, Color Plate 11-1H. **F** From Koneman EW, et al. Color Atlas and Textbook of Diagnostic Microbiology, 5th ed. Baltimore: LWW, 1997, Color Plate 11-2E; Courtesy of Becton-Dickenson Microbiology Systems, Cockeysville, MD. **G** From Koneman EW, et al. Color Atlas and Textbook of Diagnostic Microbiology, 5th ed. Baltimore: LWW, 1997, Color Plate 11-2A. **H** From Koneman EW, et al. Color Atlas and Textbook of Diagnostic Microbiology, 5th ed. Baltimore: LWW, 1997, Color Plate 11-2B. **I** From Koneman EW, et al. From Color Atlas and Textbook of Diagnostic Microbiology, 5th ed. Baltimore: LWW, 1997, Color Plate 11-2C. **J** From Koneman EW, et al. Color Atlas and Textbook of Diagnostic Microbiology, 5th ed. Baltimore: LWW, 1997, Color Plate 11-2D; Courtesy of Murex Diagnostics, Norcross, GA.

Figure 7-4: **A-1** From Freundlich IM, Bragg DG. A Radiologic Approach to Diseases of the Chest, 2nd ed. Baltimore: LWW, 1997, page 462. **A-3** From Damjanov I. Histopathology: A Color Atlas and Textbook. Baltimore: LWW, 1996, page 135. **B-1** From Freundlich IM, Bragg DG. A Radiologic Approach to Diseases of the Chest, 2nd ed. Baltimore: LWW, 1997, page 456. **C-1** From Rubin E, Farber JL. Pathology, 3rd ed. Baltimore: LWW, 1999, page 614. **D-1** From Rubin E, Farber JL. Pathology, 3rd ed. Baltimore: LWW, 1999, page 613. **E-1** From Freundlich IM, Bragg DG. A Radiologic Approach to Diseases of the Chest, 2nd ed. Baltimore: LWW, 1997, page 441. **E-2** From Burton GRW, Engelkird PG. Microbiology for the Health Sciences, 7th ed. Baltimore: LWW, 2004, page 101. **E-3** From Koneman EW, et al. Color Atlas and Textbook of Diagnostic Microbiology, 5th ed. Baltimore: LWW, 1997, Color Plate 16-1A; Courtesy of Health and Education Resources, Inc, Bethesda, MD.

Figure 7-5: **A** From Collins J, Stern EJ. Chest Radiology: The Essentials. Philadelphia: LWW, 1999, page 159. **B** From Collins J, Stern EJ. Chest Radiology: The Essentials. Philadelphia: LWW, 1999, page 159. **C** From Freundlich IM, Bragg DG. A Radiologic Approach to Diseases of the Chest, 2nd ed. Baltimore: LWW, 1997, page 470. **D** From Rubin E, Farber JL. Pathology, 3rd ed. Baltimore: LWW, 1999, page 607. **E** From Burton GRW, Engelkird PG. Microbiology for the Health Sciences, 7th ed. Baltimore: LWW, 2004, page 4. **F** From Koneman EW, et al. Color Atlas and Textbook of Diagnostic Microbiology, 5th ed. Baltimore: LWW, 1997, Color Plate 17-1H. **G** From Koneman EW, et al. Color Atlas and Textbook of Diagnostic Microbiology, 5th ed. Baltimore: LWW, 1997, Color Plate 17-1C.

H From Koneman EW, et al. Color Atlas and Textbook of Diagnostic Microbiology, 5th ed. Baltimore: LWW, 1997, Color Plate 17-1D. **I** From Koneman EW, et al. Color Atlas and Textbook of Diagnostic Microbiology, 5th ed. Baltimore: LWW, 1997, Color Plate 17-1E. **J** From Koneman EW, et al. Color Atlas and Textbook of Diagnostic Microbiology, 5th ed. Baltimore: LWW, 1997, Color Plate 17-1A.

Figure 7-6: A From Freundlich IM, Bragg DG. A Radiologic Approach to Diseases of the Chest, 2nd ed. Baltimore: LWW, 1997, page 498. **B** From Koneman EW, et al. Color Atlas and Textbook of Diagnostic Microbiology, 5th ed. Baltimore: LWW, 1997, Color Plate 14-2E. **C** From Koneman EW, et al. Color Atlas and Textbook of Diagnostic Microbiology, 5th ed. Baltimore: LWW, 1997, Color Plate 14-2D. **D** From Koneman EW, et al. Color Atlas and Textbook of Diagnostic Microbiology, 5th ed. Baltimore: LWW, 1997, Color Plate 14-2F.

Figure 7-7: A From Sarosi GA, Davis SF. Fungal Diseases of the Lung, 3rd ed. Baltimore: LWW, 2000, page 200. **B** From Koneman EW, et al. Color Atlas and Textbook of Diagnostic Microbiology, 5th ed. Baltimore: LWW, 1997, Color Plate 13-3E. **C** From Koneman EW, et al. Color Atlas and Textbook of Diagnostic Microbiology, 5th ed. Baltimore: LWW, 1997, Color Plate 13-3D.

Figure 7-8: A From Collins J, Stern EJ. Chest Radiology: The Essentials. Philadelphia: LWW, 1999, page 232. **B** From Burton GRW, Engelkird PG. Microbiology for the Health Sciences, 7th ed. Baltimore: LWW, 2004, page 129. **C** From Koneman EW, et al. Color Atlas and Textbook of Diagnostic Microbiology, 5th ed. Baltimore: LWW, 1997, page 1032. **D** From Burton GRW, Engelkird PG. Microbiology for the Health Sciences, 7th ed. Baltimore: LWW, 2004, page 129. **E** From Koneman EW, et al. Color Atlas and Textbook of Diagnostic Microbiology, 5th ed. Baltimore: LWW, 1997, Color Plate 19-5E.

Figure 7-9: A From Collins J, Stern EJ. Chest Radiology: The Essentials. Philadelphia: LWW, 1999, page 98. **B (top)** From Koneman EW, et al. Color Atlas and Textbook of Diagnostic Microbiology, 5th ed. Baltimore: LWW, 1997, page 1034. **C** From Koneman EW, et al. Color Atlas and Textbook of Diagnostic Microbiology, 5th ed. Baltimore: LWW, 1997, Color Plate 19-5F. **D** From Koneman EW, et al. Color Atlas and Textbook of Diagnostic Microbiology, 5th ed. Baltimore: LWW, 1997, page 1034; Courtesy of G. D. Roberts.

Figure 7-10: A From Sarosi GA, Davis SF. Fungal Diseases of the Lung, 3rd ed. Baltimore: LWW, 2000, page 51. **B** From Koneman EW, et al. Color Atlas and Textbook of Diagnostic Microbiology, 5th ed. Baltimore: LWW, 1997, page 1029. **C** From Koneman EW, et al. Color Atlas and Textbook of Diagnostic Microbiology, 5th ed. Baltimore: LWW, 1997, Color Plate 19-5C. **D-1** From Sarosi GA, Davis SF. Fungal Diseases of the Lung, 3rd ed. Baltimore: LWW, 2000, page 53. **D-2** From Koneman EW, et al. Color Atlas and Textbook of Diagnostic Microbiology, 5th ed. Baltimore: LWW, 1997, page 1029.

Figure 7-11: A From Daffner RH. Clinical Radiology: The Essentials, 2nd ed. Baltimore: LWW, 1999, page 127. **B** From Damjanov I. Histopathology: A Color Atlas and Textbook. Baltimore: LWW, 1996, page 137. **C** From Koneman EW, et al. Color Atlas and Textbook of Diagnostic Microbiology, 5th ed. Baltimore: LWW, 1997, page 1005. **D** From Koneman EW, et al. Color Atlas and Textbook of Diagnostic Microbiology, 5th ed. Baltimore: LWW, 1997, Color Plate 19-1C.

Figure 7-12: A From Sarosi GA, Davis SF. Fungal Diseases of the Lung, 3rd ed. Baltimore: LWW, 2000, page 98. **B** From Marler LM, Siders JA, Allen SD. Direct Smear Atlas. Baltimore: LWW, 2001, page 193. **C** From Koneman EW, et al. Color Atlas and Textbook of Diagnostic Microbiology, 5th ed. Baltimore: LWW, 1997, Color Plate 19-6C. **D** From Koneman EW, et al. Color Atlas and Textbook of Diagnostic Microbiology, 5th ed. Baltimore: LWW, 1997, Color Plate 19-6D.

Figure 7-13: A From Collins J, Stern EJ. Chest Radiology: The Essentials. Philadelphia: LWW, 1999, page 238. **B** From Koneman EW, et al. Color Atlas and Textbook of Diagnostic Microbiology, 5th ed. Baltimore: LWW, 1997, Color Plate 20-7H.

Figure 8-1: B Modified from Dudek RW. High Yield Histology, 3rd ed. Baltimore: LWW, 2004, page 34. **C** Modified from Dudek RW. High Yield Histology, 3rd ed. Baltimore: LWW, 2004, page 35.

Index

Page numbers in *italics* denote figures; those followed by a t denote tables